THE EVENT OF PSYCHOPOETICS

The Event of Psychopoetics overviews and investigates the notion of *psychopoetics*, a sociopsychological event that involves re-creative slips and that emerges under certain cultural conditions and power relations in the context of everyday interaction and through certain modes of dialoguing and conversing.

This transdisciplinary text takes the reader through the thought processes of Deleuze, Guattari, Agamben, Maffesoli, Foucault, Butler, Haraway, and Braidotti, among others, addressing debates that are integral to the critique of psychology and its devices of subjectivization and normalization. Garcia takes a unique approach by reflecting on how psychopoetics contrasts institutionalized dialogues, while constantly emphasizing the generative and transformative potency of social worlds effectuated in the impetuous play of poetics. The book combines the rigor of academic research with the creative display of ideas that open diverse, suggestive lines of reflection on everyday interlocution and its possibilities of reinvention, modes of social existence, and the relation between subjectivity and the designs of power.

A truly unique reading experience, this book is ideal for students, instructors, and researchers in the fields of philosophy, social psychology and sociological thought, discourse studies, literary theory, and cultural analysis.

Raúl Ernesto García is a tenured, full-time professor/researcher in the Faculty of Psychology at the Universidad Michoacana de San Nicolás de Hidalgo in Morelia, México. His general areas of research include theory and critique of cultural and discursive processes and subjectivization; and studies of the concept of dialogue and conversation and their current utilization in interventive apparatuses of the psychological complex. García has also published numerous specialized articles and book chapters on the aforementioned topics, as well as the book *El diálogo en descomposición* (2008), an essay on the emergence and transformations of the concept of *dialogue* in philosophical milieus and social thought.

Concepts for Critical Psychology: Disciplinary Boundaries Re-thought
Series editor: Ian Parker

Developments inside psychology that question the history of the dis-cipline and the way it functions in society have led many psychologists to look outside the discipline for new ideas. This series draws on cutting edge critiques from just outside psychology in order to complement and question critical arguments emerging inside. The authors provide new perspectives on subjectivity from disciplinary debates and cultural phe-nomena adjacent to traditional studies of the individual.

The books in the series are useful for advanced level undergraduate and postgraduate students, researchers and lecturers in psychology and other related disciplines such as cultural studies, geography, literary theory, philosophy, psychotherapy, social work and sociology.

Most recently published titles:

THE EVENT OF PSYCHOPOETICS

Imagination and The Rupture of Psychology

Raúl Ernesto García
Translated by Paul C. Kersey

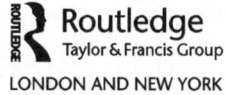

Routledge
Taylor & Francis Group

LONDON AND NEW YORK

First published 2022
by Routledge
2 Park Square, Milton Park, Abingdon, Oxon OX14 4RN

and by Routledge
605 Third Avenue, New York, NY 10158

Routledge is an imprint of the Taylor & Francis Group, an informa business

British Library Cataloguing-in-Publication Data
A catalogue record for this book is available from the British Library

Library of Congress Cataloging-in-Publication Data
Names: García, Raúl Ernesto, 1967- author.
Title: The event of psychopoetics: imagination and the rupture of psychology / Raúl Ernesto García; translated by Paul C. Kersey.
Description: Milton Park, Abingdon, Oxon; New York, NY: Routledge, 2022. | Includes bibliographical references and index.
Identifiers: LCCN 2021008976 (print) | LCCN 2021008977 (ebook) | ISBN 9780367654023 (hardback) | ISBN 9780367654016 (paperback) | ISBN 9781003129295 (ebook)
Subjects: LCSH: Poetry–Therapeutic use. | Psychotherapy and literature.
Classification: LCC RC489.P6 G37 2022 (print) | LCC RC489.P6 (ebook) | DDC 616.89/1656–dc23
LC record available at https://lccn.loc.gov/2021008976
LC ebook record available at https://lccn.loc.gov/2021008977

ISBN: 978-0-367-65402-3 (hbk)
ISBN: 978-0-367-65401-6 (pbk)
ISBN: 978-1-003-12929-5 (ebk)

DOI: 10.4324/9781003129295

Typeset in Bembo
by MPS Limited, Dehradun

CONTENTS

FOREWORD

It is a bold book that proclaims itself to be an 'event', but this is such a book, more or less. It is less in the sense that it modestly positions itself in the context of already socially-historically-constructed critiques of psychology. In this respect it operates as a clear and witty review of ideas about language in and against the discipline, ideas that interrupt and so 'rupture' ostensibly smooth narratives about the human subject in psychology textbooks and countless repetitive research articles based on those narratives. This book is thus a kind of 'counter-text', and a 'counter-narrative', even what the historian and philosopher Michel Foucault once commended as a form of 'counter-memory'. Raúl Ernesto García helps us remember what has been said so that we can say it better, radicalise it, put it to work.

And then, at the same time, the book is even more than it would first seem to be. This is not so much because it takes us beyond the many claims by critical psychologists to have at long last cracked open the discipline, found a way forward, a way out, but because the book draws attention to what must take place for those cracks to be really opened up, for a genuine alternative to emerge. The key here lies not in the claim that one particular event will do the trick, but that each intervention must have the boldness of approach, the radical energy to be an event. We are looking here not for one event – like a book in a series on concepts for critical psychology, say – but for an invitation, incitement to readers sick of the stultifying banal representations of human beings as they are now to have the courage to themselves intervene. The promise of this book is that there could be many events, that there must be two, three, many events for us to build something more worthwhile.

The book shows us that we need to really take seriously the 'turn to language' in psychology that gave rise to so many methodological innovations concerned with 'discourse' and 'narrative'. Instead of attempting to adapt those methodological innovations to the needs of the discipline of psychology, turning them into mere 'methods', steps in an analysis that can be faithfully and unthinkingly followed by students and researchers. Instead of then falling into the trap of searching inside the head of the individuals for the source of the meanings we describe in our analysis – turning the methodological innovations back into psychology – we need to move, as it were, 'sideways'. We take a sideways, horizontal move into the domain of poetics. This then also enables us to answer, in a quite different way the concerns of those critical psychologists who argued for the 'repopulation' of psychology, for the creative repopulation of experiments that had been evacuated of actual human beings. One could even say that it is, in this respect, progressively 'post-human'.

This book's imaginative argument for 'psychopoetics' charts a new domain of work that is not obedient to the traditional psychological demand that we simply describe regularities in behaviour or try to open the brain-box and search for cognitive mechanisms. Neither is it in line with simple humanistic objections to behaviourism or cognitivism – a so-called 'third force' in psychology that quickly turned itself into another version of psychology, one more attuned to confession than to discipline. Nor, it should be noticed, is it in line with normative psychoanalytic approaches that delve into the unconscious and thus replicate again and again what psychoanalysts expect to find inside the mind. Again, we move sideways in this book, to the idea that we must create, intervene, disturb the boundaries between the inside and the outside of the human subject, and the boundaries between the inside and the outside of the discipline.

There is also something surreal about this book at moments, something that reminds us that this is from Mexico, 'outwith' Western psychology, even decolonising it. *The Event of Psychopoetics: Imagination and the Rupture of Psychology* gives us practical playful creative examples of how we can be outwith the discipline and the individual, developing research that addresses the 'psyche' while also doing justice to what is 'poetic' in human life, academic, professional or not.

Ian Parker, University of Manchester

PART I

The devices of psychology and their critique

1

THE *PSYCHOLOGICAL COMPLEX* AND CRITICAL ALTERNATIVES IN PSYCHOLOGY

The problem of intervention in psychology

The idea of *intervention* constitutes one of the most important conceptual projections and practices in any area of the application of psychology. Psychological intervention entails performing certain actions that affect or influence others with a certain intention to transform the subjective and intersubjective systems or apparatuses of interpersonal relations. In other words, it involves an attempt to exert a certain influence upon others in order to achieve certain effects. *Intervening* in psychology thus means participating in an issue, problem, or conflict. It interposes a criterion associated with a set of actions directed towards mediating or interceding, from psychology, in a situation that is problematic for the subjects involved. In this sense, psychological intervention constitutes an *intromission* into people's internal affairs. Using some word play, we can think that intervening through psychology means interceding in the issues, problems, or conflicts of individuals with the goal of fulfilling a mission. From this perspective, intervention is the antonym of abstention (though "abstaining" can at times also be a way of intervening). It assumes that a process of enquiry and investigation (diagnosis) is a necessary aspect that accompanies the interventive participation itself. In effect, psychological intervention presupposes a certain assessment of both the *problematic* intersubjective situations of which the individual is object and, at some point, of the individual particularities of the subject involved. Douglas Bernstein and Michael Nietzel affirm, for example, that clinical intervention

DOI: 10.4324/9781003129295-1

describes "the explicit and professional attempts of psychologists to change the behaviour of their clients in a desired direction (.) 'intervening' in a literal sense means 'entering the action'; interceding or interfering".[1]

Therefore, the psychological problematics into which interventive activity enters are diverse. We speak, for example, of difficulties in establishing and developing interpersonal relations; of subjects' feelings of anxiety, tension, or insatisfaction with their own behaviour or attitudes; of certain perceptions of the world and oneself; or of the inability to function adequately in certain areas of life; among other issues. This is why, in everyday psychological practice, *intervention* is related – according to the case – to such objectives as: modifying behaviours, contributing to achieving a certain understanding of some issue or another, developing personal resources in order to assimilate or confront a given situation or conflict, fostering the stability and emotional *wellbeing* of individuals, groups, or families, transforming a person's self-image, that of others, or of the world in which she/he lives, modifying lifestyles, fomenting *restructurings of personality*, and promoting the acquisition and development of social abilities and competencies, among others; none of which, evidently, can be achieved in the absence of establishing certain encounters, certain relations of interlocution or communication, dialogues, and conversations of diverse character between intervener and intervened.

The *interventive* encounters in the doings of psychology develop in this relation an epistemological, ethical, and political role that is subordinated to strategies of social *normalization and harmonization* drawn by the vectors of knowledge, power, and subjection of contemporary institutions. This means that over the course of the different forms of intervention in psychology, what often appears, in specific terms of utilization, is the resource of the interpersonal encounter – as revealed in the declarations from the onset of the intervention itself – as a medium for the *transformative action* of the other (by, for instance, producing certain knowledge, reproducing values, and/or modifying attitudes, behaviours, or discourses) always from a certain position of the professional *authority* of the psychologist or intervener, whether in the clinical, educational, psychosocial, community, or workspace. In one way or another, the intervener acts specifically on individuals or groups where, sooner or later, face-to-face interaction becomes essential and, in consequence, the moment of the encounter, specific dialogue, or conversation, emerges as a resource that, tacitly or explicitly, becomes a fundamental element. In any case, the principle theoretical models that have habitually sustained the work of psychological intervention – above all in psychotherapy – come from the so-called psychodynamic models, from systemic conceptions, from behavioural and cognitive-behavioural focuses, and from the so-called humanistic currents and phenomenological-existential models with their respective practical derivations and articulations.

Having said this, we can affirm that in the professional context, *psychotherapy, orientation,* and *training* are the practices that have been constituted as some of the most important modalities of psychological intervention today. Of course, other forms of strictly *psychosocial* intervention exist, including such procedures as applying preventive programmes, consultations, institutional orientation, the so-called crisis intervention, creating self-help groups, and urban social action, among others.

Reaching any clear technical distinction among these varied forms of psychological intervention is difficult because the complexity of the *objects* approached often leads the intervener to develop diverse, flexible actions. Moreover, the conceptual foundations of all the variants of intervention emerged from more-or-less similar theoretical sources. Thus, for example, C.H. Patterson states that there are no real differences between the fields of *psychological orientation* and *psychotherapy,* and that "the difficulty in establishing a separation among them begins as soon as one confronts the definitions offered by distinct authors in this regard that, due to their similarities, can be equally accepted and considered valid for psychotherapy and, at the same time, for psychological orientation".[2] Nonetheless, it is possible to profile a certain specificity for each form of psychological intervention by, precisely, contrasting them according to diverse criteria, including the central receivers, the institutional contexts in which they are developed, or the type of problems to be confronted.

Traditionally, *psychotherapy,* in its diverse variants, is applied to subjects who *suffer* from or are affected by psychological *disintegrations* that involve the notion of dysfunctionality (to a greater or lesser degree and in one form or another). This often means the presence of emotional and/or behavioural *disorders that exceed a subject's possibilities of self-regulation.* Therefore, the people who are susceptible to psychotherapeutic influence include all those individuals who have not lost a certain awareness of the world and of themselves, but who present difficulties – greater or smaller in degree – in realizing the relative capacity of self-determination and independent adjustment to vital conjunctures; that is, "difficulties in achieving a certain type of, more-or-less conscious, more-or-less active, and more-or-less volitional, self-regulation in daily co-existence".[3] But psychotherapy also tends to be associated with a context and medical spirit related to the attempt to recover the people's *mental health* that often supposes striving to attain an assumed state of affective *wellbeing* and adequate functioning in their surroundings. Psychotherapy can go on for months or even years, and, without doubt, can provoke deep, stable reactions in the person. Psychotherapy – Dionisio Zaldívar Pérez affirms – "is a process of significations in which those events or situations that were once neutral for the subject [and] unrelated to her/his problematics and disorders, come to make sense, are learned in all their signification in the framework of the procedure".[4] Psychotherapy has the possibility to develop a specific relation (a series of encounters and interlocutions) that can promote what Alexander called a *corrective emotional experience*,[5] and can be made to transit through phases or stages in accordance with the objectives established and the contents to be worked on.[6]

The *psychological orientation* is commonly used with *functional* people who present *problems related to projecting their potential*. This orientation is applied predominantly in non-medical, institutional contexts and from a conceptual perspective focused more on the notion of *personal development* than that of "mental health". The types of problems that this approach deals with are almost always educational or professional in nature and related to decision-making processes. This orientation usually requires a short-term process (a few sessions or encounters) and the relation it fosters has a much lower emotional charge. Thus, Tyler defines this approach as "the facilitating process of prudent choices, on which the final perfectioning of the person depends".[7] The goals of this orientation include defining and clarifying the problems that the subject presents, facilitating the decision-making process in relation to it, contributing to develop the person's capacity to deal with or overcome operative obstacles in their perspective of social insertion and, in some cases, reassess aspirations and strategies in relation to her/his real possibilities and to the specific contexts in which she/he interacts. It is often considered important, during this orientation process, to develop a *communicative relationship* that guarantees *respect* for the subject's discourses, values, and motivations though, of course, this does not impede the possibility that subjects may be coerced (through informative saturation, for example) to redirect their efforts towards *developmental* goals or objectives closer to the social requirements of adaptation and normalization.

The so-called *psychological training* emerges from the conception that a certain inadequate personal functioning is not based on some "pathology" or another but, rather, on a deficit of social abilities that can be acquired and/or developed. It seeks to surmount the limitations of the traditional clinical model that centres on *illness* and tacitly promotes a relational space of a receptive-passive nature that, it is said, often undervalues the ideas of prevention, promoting health, and psychological development, by omitting other options of interpretation and action related to the *dysfunctions* of the individuals so treated. Dionisio Zaldívar Pérez observes that

> The lack of abilities can lead many subjects to present serious social deficits as a consequence of a reduced social competence that, in some cases, is expressed in such disorders as depression, alcoholism, [and] social phobias, to mention but a few, and that can also be manifested in what various authors have called social anxiety.[8]

Psychological intervention in the modality of training strives to consider, at all times, the socio-environmental context and the specific conditions of life in which the subject acts. In fact, through the "competence model" it attempts to foster changes in the contexts that sustain certain social behaviours – that is, *changes in institutions* or *communities* – and to develop actions implemented to increase the *personal competencies* of individuals: "This model, in its approach to health, inspires two basic objectives: 1) fomenting individual competence; and 2) developing competent communities and organizations".[9] Thus, the notion of training viewed from this angle involves the participation not only of subjects (who, of their own will must solve specific problems by applying personal abilities, skills, and resources that they acquire and project), but also of the social support networks (family, groups, institutions) to which they have access, and networks or systems of specialized professional support (psychologists, psychiatrists) when dealing with problems whose peculiarities demand it. Subjects may, then, appropriate the resource of *personal competence* when in their context there exist the productive activities and experiences of learning and developing the abilities and skills required to assume and resolve the demands they receive from the environment. In this logic, specialists deploy, for example, training programmes in "problem-solving", "techniques for confronting stress", specific "social abilities", or "abilities for coping with the transitions in the development of the life-cycle", among others.

In terms of *psychosocial intervention*, authors speak of multiple, diverse procedures directed towards promoting changes in various social and institutional systems and areas at the group and community levels. G.N. Fischer, for example, posits that the broad fields of intervention in social psychology focus on intercultural relations, *social cognition*, problems and phenomena of groups, institutional organization and its avatars, the social environment, and personal relations in distinct symbolic spaces.[10] But, psychosocial intervention also has to do with the conservation, consolidation, functioning, and development of socio-productive and control systems that run from increasing efficiency at work, elaborating public opinion, and influencing the mood of different social groups, to legitimizing and/or optimizing specific community practices and networks, and transforming the cultural environment. Some concrete interventive methods of psychosocial character consist in exercising *prevention* (that is, organizing preventive *programmes* directed at some target population to provide community skills, abilities, and resources for confronting sociocultural or environmental problems), *consulting* and *institutional assessment*, the so-called *crisis intervention* (*i.e.*, therapeutic actions of short duration or rapid orientation with limited objectives focused on attending to subjects in a state of *vulnerability* in situations of emergency), creating *therapeutic communities* and *self-help groups*, *urban social action* (*i.e.*, organizing community movements that present claims of a diverse character or enter into social negotiations in the pursuit of shared interests), among others.[11]

Psychosocial intervention is thus associated with the search for better *quality of life*, collective *wellbeing*, and the development of knowledge and competencies (that is, enhanced *functioning*) by the members of the intervened community, organization, or group. It presupposes *explanations*, *predictions*, and *evaluations* of the exercises conducted.

> *Psychosocial intervention* – Encarnación Nouvilas Pallejá points out – is clearly the path that the application of social psychology must follow to achieve the goals of reducing social problems [and] improving quality of life, or people's wellbeing or lives in general. For example, it might attempt to increase respect among peers at an educational centre by managing conflicts among students, or to foment preventive health behaviours and measures. In a sanitary context, it might try to reduce the probability that [people] develop disorders that can lead to disease, or risk factors for health.[12]

Psychosocial intervention, then, can span distinct *domains of analysis*: "intrapersonal", "interpersonal", "group", and "societal",[13] by continuing through different stages or steps of execution in many areas social of life.

The notion of *psychological intervention* (in its predominant technical applications) articulates its action through the deployment of an epistemological and political mandate that entails, more-or-less explicitly, the mission to *control* the subjects in whom it intervenes. Indeed, although psychologists may ponder certain forms of *ethicity* in the different devices of psychological intervention, the entire process continues from a starting point that consists in a *violence of classification*[14] imposed upon the intervened subject. Quite naturally, a whole series of discourses and behaviours can be discerned in the subject which are then scored as, for example, "inadequate", "disordered", or "abnormal", based on a codification provided by the dominant apparatuses of knowledge-power. Professional interveners, usually acritical and unaware of the political character of their activity, design and execute actions and programmes of *psychological work* – congruent, above all, with the *adaptive* logic of standardization – that influence, in one way or another, the subject's problematics, but that necessarily constrict their expression to the milieu of the *interventive encounter* by virtue of which it contributes to consolidating the active character of their own *subjection*. Ultimately, even in the nuances and complexities of the interventive exercise, the intervener acts *on* the subject through an attitude of a certain conceptual and operative *indivisibility* that predisposes, beforehand, any encounter with that subject (encounters that must proceed following the canons and conditions established by the professional format itself, however innovative and flexible that may be) and that, therefore, somehow predisposes all understanding with respect to the subject, and her/his perceptions and conflicts.[15]

In the reflexive line proposed by Nikolas Rose,[16] one can comprehend that the *disciplinarization* of psychology is constitutively related to the transformations of rationality and the technologies of political power since the late 19th century; a moment at which *government* was exercised to guarantee, insofar as possible, *physical* and *mental normality* and the *wellbeing* of citizens in a strategic project that pretended the formation and regulation of the *intimate* or *private* lifeways of workers, fathers, mothers, and people in general. Power codified as the *State* deploys its actions as part of a broad programme of guiding behaviour through diverse social authorities. *Psi knowledge* and its technical procedures were utilized from the start to promote and consolidate exercises of self-control or self-conduction of individuals in accordance with the norms of social co-existence and development. Psychology became, inevitably, a *technology of subjectivation*; a rational practice of subjection applied socially in the name of virtue, happiness, efficiency, health, grace, or self-dominion.

Psychology, psychiatry, psychotherapy, and their related derivations and technologies (the *psychological complex*) appear and function in relation to a wider field of systems of social, political, and ethical regulation at a concrete historical moment of western civilization, and have performed a key role in configuring the criteria, perceptions, and practices of people with respect to themselves in the present. Ángel Gordo López defines the *psychological complex* as "the set of networks and connections between theories and practices that psychological knowledge and government elaborate and implement".[17] In this ambit we find fundamental works, including those by Rose himself.[18]

From proposals of this kind, one comes to comprehend that the way in which subjective life and the distinct forms of interaction among people are today conceived as being related to the administrative politics of modernity and truths long-supported by the dominant scientific institutions. The psychological complex extends and reorganizes positive prescriptions, practices, and techniques of adaptation, conflict reduction, and the development of distinct social groups, always within a determined conception or cosmovision of reality and of social life itself, by virtue of which the *interventive* moment becomes unappealable and, in fact, is naturalized.

The encounter of psychological intervention tends to be materialized through (or with the concomitant participation of) a series of technical measures or instruments, diverse objects, and specific spaces that must not be seen as simple accessories of the exercise of interventive interlocution but, rather, as elements and aspects that contribute substantially to the very constitution of encounters of this kind. Interlocution takes on body to the extent to which it is constructed by this entire, changing set of apparatuses and objects that make the interview produced a practice of a profound *instrumental* condition. How is the interventive encounter in psychology to be developed if not, for example, through (*and as a derivation of*) some *tests* or diverse diagnostic or experimental or resources, *suitable* furnishings (though minimal), or a space with certain material conditions prepared previously for this task? This is how encounters of intervention come to involve not only a discursive moment, or one of spoken language, but to take on a technical-practical-material character. Its existence and development are inseparable from the heterogeneous, complex, and changing entanglement of artefacts, elements, objects, and procedures that make up *circuits of interventive activity*, together with the utilization of theories or systems that are more-or-less consistent in terms of explaining and interpreting what transpires.

Nikolas Rose suggests that there exist conditions of construction of meaning that go beyond both the speaking subject and what is said. This is, of course, applicable to the encounter that unfolds during psychological intervention. Said encounter articulates distinct discourses as systems of signification that are simultaneously associated with complex technical devices of a practical-material order to *generate the precise physical-symbolic places* for achieving such forms of interpersonal relation. A key aspect, then, of the definition of the interventive encounter would include not only w*hat is said* but also the material conditions and networks that permit a certain specialized enunciation – in technological terms.

In effect, psychological intervention promotes encounters that operate as gears of the technological device involved, which brings into play not only diverse thoughts, affects, and attitudes on the part of the inter-locutors, but also a set of abilities, skills, and competencies on the part of those responsible for the intervention that, upon intertwining with some other artefacts or techniques of specific inscription, perform, on the one hand, the function of *fabricating* diagnostic categories or forms of under-standing with respect to the subject (with their more-or-less subtle or crass consequent effects of manipulation, control, and prescription of the subject's perceptions, sentiments, and actions); and, on the other, the function of *ordering* said subject by framing, producing, or *reproducing* it in terms of subjection. With this, *a certain mode of existence* is installed and naturalized that is susceptible to being thought and treated in a certain way by the psychological complex itself. Intervention uses the encounter as a heterogeneous assemblage for directing behaviours, criteria, and sensibilities towards the ambits of reproductive normalization.

Despite its diversity of distinct modalities, the interventive exercise somehow entails installing *new truths* through a kind of act of symbolic violence. It assumes a process of interpersonal relation oriented towards the *inclusion* of the intervened subject (or perhaps her/his *reclusion*) in a pre-established model of social functioning that contains and extends its own arguments of validity and legitimacy, its *evidences*, its dominant convictions, its institutions, and its devices of justification and con-firmation. However, intervention also *seduces* because it problematizes and mobilizes proposals and activities that are forged and propagated as *solutions* to people's difficulties, sufferings, or *requirements*. The inter-ventive exercise sometimes entails persuasions, negotiations, and calcu-lations. It designs schemes of perception that permit the *visualization* of certain entities, *facts*, or *conflicts* according to specific patterns or values. It utilizes a more-or-less specific language to designate situations or ideas in special terms or vocabularies, and codifies them according to the objective or goals of the intervention itself. It tends to establish and extend *con-nections of influence* and alliances with other networks of institutional work (such as medical services, educational or study settings, workplaces, etc.) to achieve broader coverage in *attending* to the difficulties it treats. But what actually occurs is that any apparatus of intervention, articulated at different moments by *ad hoc* encounters and interactions maintains (or intensifies with greater sophistications) the separation between the in-tervener possessor of supposed theoretical-techniques capacities, and the intervened subject, whose primordial function continues to be – regardless of how "democratized" the apparatus of intervention may be – that of offering data, generating evidences, and constituting her/himself in an *object* of the pre-established disciplinary inscriptions, procedures, and activities of control. What also happens quite frequently is that the social situation of the intervention *is naturalized*; that is, people often, sooner or later, become *docile* before the interventive work; the psychological subject is finally captured by those apparatuses of reproduction.

These types of tensions, seen in a specific setting, are evaluated, for example, in the work of Erica Burman, who comments:

> Questions of power are inevitably linked to therapeutic models and processes (...). Power is neither introduced [into] nor eliminated from therapeutic processes but, rather, is implicated in what therapy does and represents. The attention I have lent to the way in which therapist[s] exercise power (either by defining the terms of interpretation or positioning themselves as being better-informed) should not be interpreted as wresting merit from the process of therapy. Nor does it necessarily reflect the demand to see the session as feminist. I sustain that power is an inevitable characteristic of therapy. Perhaps the fact that this is a feminist therapy makes the questions of power more exposed. What should, at least, be made clear is that power is not monolithic, and that multiple positions emerge [from] its fragmentation and diversity of manifestations.[19]

Psychological intervention contributes to *psychologizing* various social spaces and practices because its influence marks ways of thinking, configuring, and organizing proposals, and of disseminating and *applying* truths regarding people themselves. This process of *psychologization* gradually determines the types of *psychological problems* that the professional authorities themselves say they attend and resolve in correspondence with *governmental* activities of social administration and regulation.[20] This is not to say, however, that this psychologization of social spaces imposes a unique theoretical version of the subject. Quite to the contrary, the different knowledges of psychology and its constant interventive experience guarantee interminable questionings with respect to *being a person* and to the personal characteristics of individuals. But as Nikolas Rose explains, all that variability in the psychological ways of *composing* people is converted into a key aspect for displaying power itself through the psychological complex, because this makes it possible to unite and deal with diverse concerns and difficulties in a complex network of spaces, discourses, practices, and techniques that not only *produce* but also legitimize, disseminate, and utilize *psychological truths*.

In this process, distinct fields of social life emerge as areas of "psychological" interest. What happens is that some psychological theories or arguments or others will be related to social and institutional practices, situations, and domains by virtue of which a kind of *psychological visibility* comes to be agreed upon for their explanation and development. Thus, the production and reproduction of psychological truths function as an active process of *intervention* in people and their relations. These "psychological truths" are linked to the *practical-institutional apparatuses* of social functioning (family, work, school, etc.), whose difficulties or problems are codified (that is, rationalized and theorised) in highly-specialized terms that are also actualized; terms like "neurosis", "stress", "dementia", or "attention deficit". The key characteristic of these practical-institutional apparatuses consists in their normative propensity, which immediately detects and endures any *deviation*. It is for this reason that those apparatuses become the axis of the administrative activities of the professional authorities that, at instances of the relations of knowledge and power, can diagnose, evaluate, intervene, or arbitrate the set of events or phenomena that take place at its core.

Psychology, its procedures, and objects, obtain meaning in an articulation with the apparatuses of the regulation and administration of behaviours that, in turn, are congruent with the *systems of institutional visibility* that define the standards of intelligibility, the limits of comprehensibility and tolerance, and/or the systems of judgement for such behaviours. Theorizing with verisimilitude with respect to such categories as *intelligence, personality*, or *attitudes*, will only be possible to the degree to which such reflections are not only practicable, but also, as a basic aspect, susceptible to connecting themselves efficiently to the disciplinary demands of social institutions and their authorities. Moreover, the psychological codification of social problems and behaviours *transforms* those problems and behaviours from the very first instant by synthesizing or simplifying their heterogeneity to, convert them into more-or-less *manageable* or *manipulable* aspects in view of the pre-existing mandate of the *psychological complex* to lead and control − "for the good" − the personal expressions and development of individuals in their varied environs. The psychological complex thus offers ever more novel devices and techniques for *channelling* people, for assigning them tasks of control and development, for organizing and harmonizing their functioning in the institution and in the community. In this sense, the interventive encounter makes it possible to establish, or implant, relatively unitary spaces of explanation and deliberation of conflicts or problems, while also pre-tending to rationalize aspects of individuality, and tending to simplify, or erase, differences. In any case, it can become an instrument of support and follow-up of institutional projects for healing, for teaching, or for the social reinsertion of the people involved.

But perhaps the most important aspect is that the exercise of inter-vention contributes to governing behaviour from the moment that, im-bued with psychological terminologies and techniques, it boasts a supposed *ethical foundation* because it seeks to *recognize* the intervened subjects and works to establish and promote people's own capacity to deploy *authority* and control on themselves (that is, self-government) and, in this way, improve their potential for *development* and *wellbeing*. The interventive exercise thus establishes and foments ways of speaking, thinking, feeling, and acting that are susceptible to ongoing evaluation and administration. The intervened subjects, therefore, are exposed and open to ulterior calculations, manipulations, and violences *in the name of work with subjectivity*. They can learn to judge and value their own ex-istence, to re-signify their social life, and to operate on themselves. In truth, the interventive exercise in psychology changes the way in which people can think about themselves. It obtains a veneer of credibility because it is supported by the *scientific* knowledge and experiences that interveners offer. The interventive exercise leads subjects to re-articulate themselves with the institutional machinery and trains them for other goals of development, pondered in terms of psychological qualities and capacities for relating to others.

From psychology and its dominions, the exercise of intervention is constituted as a practice of relatively stable subjection, a device for the fabrication of meanings that produce and reproduce certain forms of experience through the activation of some vocabulary or other, systems of judgement, modes of visualization, and norms, all directed towards achieving interactive efficiency and the organized and predictable func-tioning of people in their surroundings. The exercise of intervention generates problematizations with respect to the different ways in which the intervened subjects can reflect upon themselves, always in relation to their specific sociohistorical and material conditions of existence. But in all cases, we are dealing here with a practice that seeks, more-or-less consistently, to achieve the goal of social regulation; that is, a *technology* of normalization and a rationality marked by the strategic missions of *government*.

The exercise of intervention, performed in any of the established formats of psychological work, tends to *help* people *solve* problems or situations of crisis. It serves as *a guide* for a functional or *conscious* life, and contributes to designing people's feelings, aspirations, and ways of thinking and acting as a function of values or objectives that are deemed *desirable*, all at the instances of the *authorised* condition of the professionals involved. The interventive exercise, therefore, sets out to fulfil a kind of *promise* sustained upon determined ideals, goals, or prescriptions. It constitutes an important exercise in the circuits of social *ordering*, leading Óscar Daza Díaz to observe that:

> We live in a society where psychology has the role of tutor. The psychologist is the 'expert' that orients children towards their vocation and participates in formulating study plans attuned to social demands. In businesses, it gives managers leads on how to structure the organisation, and what people to hire. In publicity, it utilises its entire scientific apparatus to convince us to consume a product or a message. In justice, it evaluates the capacities of a person before a tribunal, and the trust we can place in her/his testimonio. And, of course, in personal life it diagnoses and attempts to cure psychological diseases, or helps us overcome certain personal problems. Thus, the psychologist seems to guide the consciences of the citizens of the 20th century to the point of placing itself above them and going so far as to diagnose what is the best citizen for a given situation.[21]

The interpersonal encounter, in its condition of interventive practice by psychology with its associated technical figures, does not usually assume itself as the object of questioning and rarely reflects upon its own social function within the disciplines of the *psychological complex*. The disciplinary framework of its appearance and functioning only allows its instrumental readjustment and refinement, not its critical deconstruction or dismantling. Moreover, the interventive encounter, in its technological, *codifying*, and regulating condition, tends to develop as a device for managing social antagonisms and conflicts through that kind of *psychologization* of the life of the subjects implicated in the intervention. This is to say that it fosters attributing *psychological causes* to the understanding and resolution of the many vital and interactive situations analysed and, in this way, contributes to disintegrating alternative modes of community relations and nullifying other possibilities of collective existence. It thus tends to *pathologise* differences and dissension, deploying – subtly or rather crassly – the *imperative* of health up to its idealization, and somehow marking the presumed pattern of happiness or, at least, of a mature *conscientisation* of life's problems. The interventive exercise is not, then, an encounter free of ideological values.

> In fact – as Guillermo Rendueles affirms referring to psychotherapy – many cures are nothing more than the acquisition of a moral competence in order to comply with norms: drinking, complaining, or embittering one's neighbours are bad, and 'I am capable of not doing so' can be expressed as 'I'm cured', but better as 'I acquired moral norms', with therapists performing the role of teachers of virtue that Foucault identified.[22]

Hence, intervener and intervened need to reach a consensus on values, even as a moment prior to initiating the practice of intervention itself, because it is only on the basis of such a *homogenisation* of values that the "alliance" of work becomes possible – a therapeutic contract, for example – and the performance of the exercise is facilitated.

The critical reflection on the political implications of psychological intervention begs the question of what to do? It is necessary to leave open the question of the possibility of changing things, above all because from psychological practice, *is it possible not to intervene?* Is it possible to escape from the framework and values of "the therapeutic", the assistential, or what is useful? Is it possible from psychology to think without pondering the mission to "help one's neighbour"? Can a labour exist that is not oriented directly or indirectly to "saving" the intervened subject? Is it possible to interact with the subject without the objective of completing the *mission* of "positive change"? Perhaps there is another option. The option of imagination as instant creator of the world. Imagination with all its political and poetic condition battling the onslaughts of normalization and docile functioning; imagination as subversive word and uncommon practice of freedom. Imagination understood as a field of resistance can be converted into a form of interrupting the relations of subjection present in the interventive practice of psychology. This act of resistance is possible if we understand imagination from its instituting radicality. Perhaps we can find a way to escape from the unique voice that the different forms of intervention in which psychology frames us, of fomenting new ways of thinking and imagining our experience, creating other forms of subjectivity, and generating actions that do not serve that tangled technical web of normalization called the *psychological complex*.

Some divergent alternatives in psychological work

Theoretical-practical movements like *anti-psychiatry* and the so-called *counter-psychology*, which act in the diverse terrains of psychological intervention, configure proposals and actions that seek to impugn, in their everyday work, the dominant, normalized character of the established psychological professional apparatuses. The presentation of the term "anti-psychiatry" has been attributed to David Cooper's intellectual and political effort to *invert* the rules of the traditional psychiatric game – congruent with the interventive spirit of the *psychological complex* – and eventually be able to *interrupt* those circuits of social ordering.[23] Cooper thinks of the anti-psychiatric exercise as a kind of ongoing subversive revolution that requires its followers to renounce the forms of institutional life and the monetary and symbolic hierarchies linked to psychiatric practice that derives from power. Anti-psychiatry rejects the institution of the asylum because it constitutes a form of the totalization and control of the lives of those who are *interned*. It defends the rights of the so-called mentally ill and opposes

> the perversion of the therapeutic that entails utilising a whole arsenal of techniques, those of clinical psychiatry, that are in reality (due to their genealogy and historical development and practice) artefacts for sustaining the *status quo* and, therefore, must be destroyed, for they are pathological as brakes to change. Change that is, definitively, what all therapeutic action seeks.[24]

Counter-psychology appropriates such proposals to sharpen its criticisms of the institutionalized labour of psychologists in its different fields of social application. It calls for the dismantling of the apparatuses of normalization formed by the existing disciplines of the psychological complex in an effort to (for example) "construct, instead, truly therapeutic disciplines and knowledge. This is why it (...) prefers to place itself, more than in the critique of psychology, in critical psychology".[25] Counter-psychology strives to constitute itself as a *rupturist*, not merely *reformist*, practice with respect to those apparatuses of normalization. But this is where, in my view, an inconsistency appears that can now be glimpsed: this proposal will continue to be *reformist* as long as it continues to accept, unquestioningly – as is evident – the disciplinary exercise of *intervention itself*. I can illustrate this situation with the following caricature: someone says of a painter: "how crazy is that artist who paints pictures so different and strange, that artist breaks away from what is established"; and someone else responds: "well, that painter isn't so crazy for, in the end, if *he continues to paint pictures* he is not really breaking away from what is established". In effect, the proposals that bear the sign of anti-psychiatry and counter-psychology cannot sustain a rupturist character if they continue to be *framed* in the unscathed perspective of the interventive formulation.

The anti-psychiatry and counter-psychology movement offers an eclectic posture in relation to the technical-interventive aspect that rests upon the possibility of making certain *contributions* to labours of social-therapeutic support: it rejects the acritical acceptance of medical-psychiatric taxonomies of "mental illness", and conceives people's suffering and insanity as *vital problems* of social, interactive, or language origin that is *not conventional*.[26] It opposes the abuse of psychotropic drugs and irresponsibility in prescribing and doing research on them. It understands some psychotic breakdowns in terms of personal *journeys* that open new possibilities for new knowledge of oneself, others, and the world, that can (without the aggressions of classic psychiatry) lead, not to feelings of being lost but to a return to health. It changes the way of understanding *listening* in the apparatus of attention, such that what subjects say during interlocution is received not as expression that *informs* alleged psychiatric disfunctions in them; the aim, rather, is to listen to subjects without exercising on their words that classificatory violence of psychopathological diagnosis that separates the subject from her/his vital experiences. Nor does it support the use of a listening that focuses on exclusive interpretation. The intention is to listen attentively to subjects' utterances in their delirium or depressive ideas as a language articulated in ways that differ from the norm and to attempt – as Josep Alfons Arnau establishes – to

> help the other elaborate a critical vision of her/his experience; that
> is – he continues – a listening based on respecting the subject who
> receives therapeutic aid as a person who has not lost the capacity of
> an *intentional subject*, because she/he is still alive.[27]

During the development of dialogues and conversations with the individual, these movements reject that political act of psychiatric predetermination which seeks to catalogue and control the subject by applying pre-established technical categories and resources that, in reality, eliminate – in this view – the possibility of seeing and listening to subjects in the full complexity and specificity of the vital problems that afflict them. In addition, it pretends to focus interventive work on present and future ambits, thus pondering the *desiring* condition of the subject and, above all, fomenting the notion of *freedom* as a therapeutic resource.[28] In their conceptual development, the anti-psychiatric and counter-psychological positions posit the need to foster "cooperative relations" that go beyond the orbit and zones of influence of psychiatric-psychological institutions. David Cooper, for example, went so far as to postulate the so-called "no-psychiatry" as a way to surmount the anti-psychiatric experience.[29]

Today, various theoretical-practical approaches co-exist that can, in effect, be pondered as *alternative* proposals of contemporary psychology in their diversity[30]; formulations that generate possibilities for reflection and action, more-or-less distanced from the classic, dominant conceptions or paradigms of the work of psychology. These include orthodox psychoanalysis and its principle psychodynamic variants, the broad behavioural-cognitive perspective and its interventive derivations of a rational-emotional order, or the phenomenological-existential positions that open the way for so-called *humanist* ideas. These alternative proposals are produced from minority platforms like the so-called *ethnopsychology*, reflexive variants that seek to recover oriental cultures and values like *Hindu* or *Buddhist psychology*, Hillman's *archetypal-imaginal psychology*,[31] *narrative* variants and variants of philosophical orientation, such as psychotherapeutic possibility, the so-called *dialytic* psychotherapy or *psychodialysis*, *radical psychiatry*; *imagological psychosociology*, the *transpersonal*, *transactional*, and *gestalt* variants, and from there way to Jodorowsky's *psychomagic*,[32] *schizoanalysis*,[33] or considering the alleged *poetic* dimensions of psychotherapy.[34]

In the ambit of social psychology and sociology, diverse elaborations are being developed that question the precepts and practices of the *official knowledges* of psychology, based not only on the philosophical thought of Michel Foucault, but also on the works of diverse critical sociologists: Pierre Bourdieu, Robert Castel, Erving Goffman, and Norbert Elías, among others.[35] These proposals involve a deep pondering of the social and cultural dimensions of subjectivity, and of the processes of subjectivation in contraposition to theoretical schemes that, by making the individual subject responsible for her/his acts and expressions, avoid revealing, minimizing, or *naturalising* the role of the conditions of possibility of a systemic character in the determination of those specific manifestations. Critical thinking in the terrains of sociology and psychology is focused on terms of political complexity, the relations of the subject, the production of subjectivity, and groups with a changing social world. It opposes the tendency to artificially cleave the individual from society so as to study her/him in isolation. However:

> One of the reasons why officialist psychology has grown enormously – Fernando Álvarez Uría explains – is that acritical psychology, asocial psychology, is highly-functional for the system because, in the end, it makes subjects exclusively responsible for their luck or bad luck. In this it coincides with the individualist vision of liberals and neoliberals. If someone fails at school it is because she/he is not very intelligent or is going through a rough time, and so requires psychological support. If someone is depressed, she/he needs therapy. By reducing all dysfunctions to the order of subjectivity in no way are the institutions or established social order ever questioned. Unemployment or precarious employment is never questioned, school organization is never questioned, the social field is never questioned.[36]

The social sciences also potentiate the emergence of critical perspectives based on the so-called *linguistic turn* by virtue of which they reflect on the ways in which discursive practices construct their "objects" of study during the very process of studying them. In this sense, according to Ángel Gordo López, *British critical psychology*, discursive in nature, and interested in the dynamics of power and resistance, constitutes a fundamental reference for understanding, for example, how critical and hegemonical tendencies co-exist in the context of Spanish social psychology.[37] But in Gordo López' opinion, many of the critical perspectives that can be distinguished in Spanish social psychology today sustain a basically *reformist* condition, as do the "strong versions" of British critical psychology, and go so far as to promote the *psychologisation* of resistance; that is, a *psychologism* eager to achieve disciplinary recognition of its labours that, despite their critical standing, finds itself absorbed (in terms of peaceful co-existence, neutralization, or *redefinition*, as simple theoretical-methodological innovations) by hegemonic, institutionalized, official psychology.[38] Despite the foregoing, the so-called *critical social psychology*, in its heterogeneous avatars, both European and American,[39] still opens spaces for plural discussion related to different socio-psychological realities through a productive conjugation of open elaborations of a problematic sign, such as socio-constructionism, discourse analysis, deconstruction, post-structuralist thought, diverse feminisms and gender studies, the sociology of scientific knowledge, and *cyberculture*, among others. But it also constitutes an ample resource for the genealogical analysis of historical-social processes in their complex subjective, material, and technological entanglements. It permits thinking the social *disciplines* in their links to cultural environments beyond the narrow canons of academicism and instituted professional customs while, of course, underscoring the inescapable condition of dynamic inter-penetration between the *personal* and *political* ambits of social life and the corporal and intersubjective relations in the contemporary world.

Notes

1 Bernstein, D.; Nietzel, M. (1988) *Introducción a la psicología clínica*. Mexico: McGraw-Hill, p. 308.
2 Patterson, C.H. (1980) *Theories of counseling and psychotherapy*. New York: Harper and Row (cited by Zaldívar, D. (2001) *La intervención psicológica*. Morelia: IMCED, p. 46).
3 García, R. (1999) Psicología y psicoterapia integrales: consideraciones y perspectivas. In: *Revista Ethos Educativo IMCED* (21) 88–100, p. 97.
4 Zaldívar, D. *La intervención psicológica*. Ed. cit. p. 60.
5 See: Alexander, F.; French, T. M. (1956) *Terapéutica psicoanalítica*. Buenos Aires: Paidós.
6 See also: Zaldívar, D. (1991) *Teoría y práctica de la psicoterapia*. Havana: ENPES.
7 Cited by Zaldívar, D. *La intervención psicológica*. Ed. cit. p. 48.
8 Idem, p. 70.
9 Costa, M.; López, E. (1986) *Salud comunitaria*. Madrid: Martínez Roca, p. 109.
10 Fischer, G.N. (1992) *Campos de intervención en psicología social*. Madrid: Narcea.
11 See: Sánchez, A. (1991) *Psicología comunitaria. Bases conceptuales y operativas. Métodos de intervención*. Barcelona: PPU.
12 Nouvilas, E. Psicología social aplicada. In: Morales, F., Moya, M., Gaviria, E., Cuadrado, I. (Coords.) (2007) *Psicología social*. Madrid: McGraw-Hill, p. 777.
13 See: Sapsford, R. Domains of analysis. In: Sapsford, R., Still. A., Wetherell, M.S., Miell, D., Steven, R. (1998) *Theory and social psychology*. London: Sage, pp. 65–74.
14 See: García, A. (2007) *Desclasificados. Pluralismo lógico y violencia de la clasificación*. Barcelona: Anthropos, pp. 32–42.
15 See, for example, David Good's critical reflection in his: Aproximación a los problemas lingüísticos de los esquizofrénicos desde una perspectiva interactiva. In: Álvaro, J.L., Torregrosa, J.R., Garrido, A. (Comps.) (1992) *Influencias sociales y psicológicas en la salud mental*. Madrid: Century XXI, pp. 171–192.
16 Rose, N. (1996) *Inventing ourselves. Psychology, power and personhood*. Cambridge: Cambridge University Press.
17 Gordo, A. (2006) De la crítica al academicismo metodológico: líneas de acción contra los desalojos sociocríticos. In: Romero, J.L., Álvaro, R. (Coords.) *Antipsychologicum. El papel de la psicología académica: de mito científico a mercenaria del sistema*. Barcelona: Virus, p. 49.
18 Rose, N. (1985) *The psychological complex*. London: Routledge.

19 Burman, E. (1996) Identificación, subjetividad y poder en psicoterapia feminista. In: Gordo, A., Linaza, J.L. (Comps.) (1996) *Psicologías, discursos y poder (PDP)* Madrid: Visor, pp. 285–299 (p. 296).

20 See also: Rose, N. (1990) *Governing the soul: the shaping of private self.* London: Routledge.

21 Daza Díaz, O. (2006) El paradigma del control social en los orígenes de la psicología. In: Romero, J.L., Álvaro, R. (Coords.) *Antipsychologicum. El papel de la psicología académica: de mito científico a mercenaria del sistema.* Barcelona: Virus, p. 29.

22 Rendueles, G. (2006) Vocación psicoterapéutica y queme profesional. In: Romero, J.L., Álvaro, R. (Coords.) *Antipsychologicum. El papel de la psicología académica: de mito científico a mercenaria del sistema.* Ed. cit. pp. 250–251.

23 See: Cooper, D. (1981) *Psiquiatría y antipsiquiatría.* Barcelona: Paidós. By the same author: (1978) *La gramática de la vida. Estudio de los actos políticos.* Barcelona: Ariel. Another set of highly illustrative texts is found in: Ingleby, D. (Ed.) (1982) *Psiquiatría crítica. La política de la salud mental.* Barcelona: Crítica. For a more recent evaluation see: Arnau, J.A. (2005) Aprehender nuestra historia: las aportaciones de la antipsiquiatría vistas desde la contrapsicología. In: Romero, J., Álvaro, R. (Eds.) (2005) *Psicópolis. Paradigmas actuales y alternativos en la psicología contemporánea.* Barcelona: Kairós, pp. 283–312.

24 Arnau, J.A. (2005) Aprehender nuestra historia: las aportaciones de la antipsiquiatría vistas desde la contrapsicología. In: Romero, J., Álvaro, R. (Eds.) (2005) *Psicópolis. Paradigmas actuales y alternativos en la psicología contemporánea.* Ed. cit. pp. 287–288.

25 Idem, p. 288.

26 See, on this reflection: Szas, T (1961) *El mito de la enfermedad mental. Bases para una teoría de la conducta personal.* Buenos Aires: Amorrortu, 1994 (especially Part III. "Análisis semiótico de la conducta"; pp. 121–168).

27 Arnau, J.A. (n24) p. 301.

28 In this regard, reviewed the text by Franco Basaglia (1982) Rompiendo el circuito de control. In: Ingleby, D. (Ed.) *Psiquiatría crítica. La política de la salud mental.* Ed. cit. pp. 236–246.

29 See: *Ajoblanco* (1978) Interview with David Cooper. *Ajoblanco* (30) Barcelona (Cited by Arnau, J.A. (n24) p. 305).

30 See: Romero, J., Álvaro, R. (Eds.) (2005) *Psicópolis. Paradigmas actuales y alternativos en la psicología contemporánea.* Barcelona: Kairós.

31 Hillman, J. (1999) *Re-imaginar la psicología.* Madrid: Siruela. By the same author: (1999) *El pensamiento del corazón.* Madrid: Siruela, or: (2000) *El mito del análisis.* Madrid: Siruela.

32 Jodorowsky, A. (2006) *Psicomagia.* Mexico: Grijalbo. Also: (2001) *La danza de la realidad. Memorias.* Mexico: Grijalbo.

33 Deleuze, G., Guattari, F. (1972) *El Anti-Edipo. Capitalismo y esquizofrenia.* Barcelona: Paidós, 1998 (especially Ch. IV "Introducción al esquizoanálisis" pp. 283–392).

34 As K. Gergen himself does in a relatively recent text: (2006) *Construir la realidad. El futuro de la psicoterapia.* Barcelona: Paidós (specifically Ch. 6, entitled "La poética de la psicoterapia" pp. 173–184).

35 See: Álvarez-Uría, F. (2006) Psicología y sociología: hacia una cooperación necesaria. In: Romero, J.L., Álvaro, R. (Coords.) *Antipsychologicum. El papel de la psicología académica: de mito científico a mercenaria del sistema.* Ed. cit. pp. 13–25.

36 Idem, pp. 23–24.
37 Gordo, A. (2006) De la crítica al academicismo metodológico: líneas de acción contra los desalojos sociocríticos. In: Romero, J.L., Álvaro, R. (Coords.) *Antipsychologicum. El papel de la psicología académica: de mito científico a mercenaria del sistema.* Ed. cit. p. 44.
38 See the detailed analysis: Idem, pp. 45–55 and ss.
39 See, in this regard: González, F. (2004) La crítica en la psicología social latinoamericana y su impacto en los diferentes campos de la psicología. *Revista Interamericana de Psicología 38* (2) 351–360.

2

THE ENERGY OF *POIESIS*

In his book, *El hombre sin contenido*, Giorgio Agamben presents a series of reflections on the relation between *poiesis* and *praxis*.[1] There, he underscores that *poiesis* designates the very essence of human beings; namely, productive work, including artistic endeavours. Being human entails a poetic condition; that is, a productive condition. In *El Banquete*, Plato identified the notion of *poiesis* as creative activity in general and as a form of wisdom.[2] *Poiesis* constitutes the moment of creation and the process by virtue of which something passes from *not being* to *being*. Hence, every time something is produced, every time something is brought out of concealment and into the *light of the presence*, *poiesis* will exist, there will be *production*. Here we are dealing with the notion of *creation* in its most radical sense, its ontological sense.

Agamben, however, goes on to explain that Aristotle would later distinguish between that which by *being by nature* contains within itself its own beginning and origin of its entrance into the presence, from that other which does not contain within itself its own beginning but finds it, precisely, in the productive activity of human beings.[3] In Aristotelian terms, productive activity towards the presence (that is, *poetic* becoming) has the character of *installation in a form*; passing from *not being* to *being* means acquiring a figure, assuming a form. Thus, the *originality* of a given work alludes not only to the fact that it is unique or distinct from other works, but also signifies *proximity to the origin*. This means that the work will have a special relation with its origin: when *poiesis* enters, the work is produced in the presence of a form and, based on that form, "maintains a

DOI: 10.4324/9781003129295-2

relation of proximity with its formal beginning such that the possibility that its entrance into the presence become somehow reproducible is excluded (...)".[4]

Derived from this is the notion that wherever technique emerges, the formal beginning is simply an exterior paradigm, or mould, to which the product must be adapted, while the creative act remains in a *reproducible* state. Reproducibility (understood here "as paradigmatic relation of no proximity to the origin") is the key condition of products of technique, just as originality (or authenticity) is the key condition of *artistic* work.[5] There exists, then, a double condition of the creative activity of human beings; that is to say, two *spheres of poiesis*: one that, due to the effect of technique, is reproducible and cannot be said to be *original*; and one that is *irreproducible*, or that escapes from the repetitive action of technique.

For Aristotle, production towards the presence performed by *poiesis* has an *energetic* character of *actuality*, of *effective reality*, which implies that, upon entering into and remaining in the presence, it returns in the end to a form in which it encounters its own *culmination*, its own realization, *possessing itself in its own purpose*.[6] This production differs from that which does not possess its own purpose; that is, from production that does not involve *its own form* but exists simply in the mode of *availability*; in other words, *being-adequate-for* a production that serves as a *means to* achieve other ends. Works that result from *poiesis*, then, will have the characteristics of unrepeatability of its form and self-delineation of its purpose. Works that are a product of technique, in contrast, lack this *energetic* condition, or of *actuality*, in their own form: "as if the characteristic of *availability* ends up obfuscating their formal aspect".[7]

The present reflection on distinct exercises, encounters, and ambits of *psychological intervention* and the alleged emergence of a *poetic* dimension in them, opens a path that leads to the following line of analysis: a practice of interlocution that is *reproduced* on the basis of *technique* – for example, a set of patterns or elements that the intervener should follow while performing a psychotherapeutic dialogue more-or-less preconceived from a certain theoretical focus – can never possess itself in either form or purpose but, rather, must remain permanently in its condition of *availability*; that is, as a *means-for*. What often takes place during the exercise of psychological intervention is a dialogue or *interlocution (more-or-less) patterned by procedure*; a dialogue whose primordial characteristic consists in implicating an *availability for* – in this case – *achieving other, diverse normalising ends or goals related to "benefitting" the subject*; the character of being a *means for* obscuring the *energetic* character – or of *actuality* – of its final result under its own condition. Even those practices of intervention which pretend or propose an "open", or "non-directive", character and that develop in a continuous dynamism and progress towards the consecution of a "strategic" objective (the subject's "personal growth" or "development of personality", for example) entail a condition of *constant availability for* given the impediment that they lack *their own form*.

According to Agamben, the difference between *poiesis* and *praxis* consists, fundamentally, in that *poiesis*, which is related to a creation in the sense of *bringing into being*, has at its core the experience of producing towards the presence; that is, the event through which something passes "from not being to being, from concealment to the full light of the work".[8] *Praxis*, in contrast, which is related to *doing* but in the sense of *realizing*, has at its core the idea of a volition expressed immediately in action. Thus, the fundamental character of *poiesis* is not found in its aspect or process of practice-concrete-voluntary realization but, rather, in constituting a form of the truth understood as *unveiling*. For Aristotle, *poiesis* exists on a higher plane than *praxis*, because *poiesis* presupposes a space of freedom and importance that *praxis* does not possess.

Agamben, however, explains that what the Greeks understood as *poiesis* was understood in the Latin world as a form of *agere*; that is, "as an action that puts-into-work, an *'operari'*".[9] This *energetic* character of *poiesis*, that for the Greeks was not related directly to action but designated the key condition of *being in presence*, was transformed by the Romans into *actus* and *actualitas*, translated as "on the plane of *agere*, the voluntary production of an effect". The consequence of this in the West was that the possibility of distinguishing between *poiesis* and *praxis* faded away: "The central experience of poiesis, production towards presence, now cedes its place to the consideration of 'how'; that is, the process through which the object has been produced". This leads to a convergence or, perhaps better, "an obfuscation of the distinction between poiesis and praxis".[10] The distinction between *poiesis* and *praxis* elaborated by the Greeks stresses, precisely, that *poiesis* is not linked to the expression of one operative volition or another, and that its most important aspect was the *unveiling*, production and "the resulting aperture of a world for the existence and action of man".[11]

Any *dialogue*, conversation, or interlocution of a *technical* nature – that is, marked or oriented by some procedure of *intervention* – will accentuate the *operari*. In contrast, an encounter that generates the emergence of the *poetic* will place its accent on the *energy* entailed in passing from *not being* to *being*, on the opening of new worlds whose emergence cannot be patterned by any operative or planned volition based on the objectives to be achieved during the encounter. Thus, it is possible to recognize that a dialogue realized as part of a determined procedure in the ambit of an *activity of psychological intervention* will be an exercise that distances itself from the zone of *poiesis* to install itself in the tessitura of *praxis*. Such a dialogue constitutes an *instrument* that obeys the logic of the procedure itself, one that serves as a *means-for*, that bears within itself an *order of use* in detriment to its latent *poetic* condition; that is, in detriment to the inauguration of other worlds, to the untimely irruption of new worlds, to the unveiling of surprising (disordered) landscapes in the play of inter-locution. Perhaps the emergence of the poetic confronts in its very constitution the dismantling of any *technical authority*. Or perhaps it promotes the creative rupturing of the chain of transmissibility and comprehensibility of the dialogical exercise (more-or-less subordinated to one cultural and discursive order or another). The emergence of the poetic thus involves a kind of destruction (or a more-or-less successful *sabotage*) of the established, or traditional, transmissibility of dialogical activity to spur the *instantaneous* – transitory, mutant – *appearance* of other worlds because, as well, the temporal dimension of all *poetics* is constituted, precisely, by the *instant*.

Enunciative fertility; aperture to experience; promotion of new *forms of being*; outline of *theory* without prescriptive vocation; imbrication with the *logos* but in constant tension due to the emergence of fantasy; emotive participation; truth as *unveiling*; uselessly inventive expression; verbal enrichment; corporal and sensory language; *freedom* of the word; play of imagination; anti-utilitarianism; intensive tangle of affirmations and actions; chromatic explosion of discourse; rupture of the usual; rebellion against boredom; experience of the generating *shock* of meaning that occurs in the interlocution. This is the, still incomplete, meaning of a *psychopoetics*.

Notes

1 Agamben, G. (1998) *El hombre sin contenido*. Barcelona: Áltera, pp. 113–154.
2 See: Plato: *Diàlegs*. Barcelona: Fundació Bernat Metge. 18 Vols. 2000. *El Banquete* 196 c, d, e (Vol. VI, pp. 65–66); 197 a (p. 66); 205 b, c (pp. 78–79).
3 Agamben, G. *El hombre sin contenido*. Ed. cit. pp. 100–101.
4 Idem, p. 102.
5 Idem, pp. 102–103.
6 Idem, p. 108.
7 Idem, pp. 108–109.
8 Idem, p. 114.
9 Idem, p. 115.
10 Idem, pp. 115–118.
11 Idem, p. 119.

3

THE *POETIC DIMENSION* IN PSYCHOLOGICAL *PRAXIS*

There is an important field of analysis of the possibilities of utilizing poetic elements in the development of practices and modalities of diverse psychological interventions (in other words, broad reflections on how to think the poetic placed at the service of the doings of psychology). We can mention, for example, the interesting proposals of the so-called *psychomagia*[1] or even, from a very distant position, the assumption of a certain *poetics* of psychoanalysis by virtue of which analytical work is related to a presumed poetic condition of *psychoanalytical technique* itself.[2] Much less reflection, however, has been devoted to how the poetic can definitively break away from psychology and its mandates; that is to say, how poetic expression, in word and action, impugns, subverts, or rebels against, the prescriptions of analysis, harmonization, and/or social functionality that the apparatuses of psychology promote and impose as part of their activities of the social administration and regulation of subjectivity. From this perspective, some current expressions of the heterogeneous world of psychological practice can be reviewed.

Psychotherapy and socio-constructionism

Based on a review and analysis of some current theoretical movements that mark the recent history of psychotherapy (namely, constructivism, the systemic and relational orientation, postmodern–post-structuralist thought, and narrative focuses), Kenneth Gergen explored, from social constructionism, what he has denominated the *poetic dimension* of therapeutic communication.[3]

DOI: 10.4324/9781003129295-3

Gergen begins by conceiving the therapeutic relation as a space that must abandon, or free itself from, the set of assumptions or methods associated with consecrated theoretical orientations, or those firmly established by the grand schools of psychology. In this regard (commenting on Gergen's work), Mony Elkaïm emphasized that

> The therapist is who strives to guide patient[s] so that other voices emerge in their interior to install other forms of *conversation*. It is not about applying or verifying a preconceived truth constructed somewhere else, not the therapeutic scenario, but about conceiving the theatre of therapy as the space of a dialogue that, through its own evolution, leads the patient towards change.[4]

Gergen further points out the need to remember that the client's or subject's accounts constitute contingent constructions that do not reflect any essential nature of the problem posited; quite to the contrary, language must be assumed as a pragmatic device united with a means of relation. Moreover, it seeks to avoid centring on the notion of *subjectivity* (understood as thoughts, emotions, or imagination) associated with the unitary *person* in order to target its relational contexts, the pragmatic meanings of the discourse involved. This leads to valuing the narrative transformations that may be produced in therapy, the alternative modalities of discourse that (positively) influence the subject's real or potential relations. This means pondering the possibility of *multiple narrations* not only as a resource for substituting "stereotyped" and "deficient" stories, but also to "help client[s] maintain better relations with their peers while making the best of the riches of language or of the production of meaning".[5] Thus, Gergen vindicates from *socio-constructionism* the accumulation of conversations developed in social life because, in his judgement, they all participate in the process of generating and modifying meanings, values, forms of comprehending, and collective knowledges including, of course, identity itself and the existential plexuses involved, which derive in a "multiplicity of egos" that have the possibility of inhabiting, at one and the same time "multiple realities".

As a result, psychotherapists must be figures who contribute to *constructing* (through their special competencies and work), in relation to others, the social milieu itself in ideological, political, and moral terms. As therapists, they take on the task of *coordinating meaning* not only at the interpersonal or familiar level, but (even) as a service to such broader social environments as, for example, inter-group settings:

"Are we able to raise ourselves sufficiently above our respective party commitments" – Gergen wonders – "to foster a communication or a coordination that will allow us to live better together in a world in which groups are increasingly opposed? This is a formidable challenge." And he goes on: "How can we devote ourselves to thinking more global political problems more systematically? What genres of practices would we have to propose if we accede to participating in conversations of this kind? What types of dialogues should be addressed and how could we facilitate them?"[6]

It is in this direction that the need to "invent other dialogical configurations" through the exercise of breaking away from the cultural tradition of dialogue as *logical argumentation* is proposed, giving priority to confrontation to demonstrate the superiority of one point of view over another, according to the principle of obligatory coherence. In this regard, one proposal is to explore other potentialities of dialogue, based on the experience of the coordination of diverse realities, towards "more cooperative modalities of exchange"; that is, more active exchanges that are not subject to the principle of *unique reality*. The idea is to constantly experience new alternatives in the psychotherapeutic (*interventive*) encounter under the aegis of the explicit or implicit alliance and to deploy to this end, in effect, an art of dialogue and conversation that succeeds, moreover, in entering the concrete life of the client-subject (being transferred to the practices of relation beyond the psychotherapeutic cabinet) and extending the capacity for more functional exchanges in different areas of specific co-existence.

Constructionist psychotherapy ponders, through Wittgenstein's work, the key influence of language and of *plays of language* (that proceed according to rules) in the descriptions and explanations that are offered to others. This evokes the regulatory character of plays of language and their use in broad *forms of life* linked to specific, material actions and environments. Thus, the distinct knowledges and ways of coordinating acts of relation take on an irreducible social character. But by the same token, if by means of psychotherapeutic activity success is attained in modifying the forms of utilization of language, forms of speaking, or the displacement of contexts of use is achieved, then – Gergen argues – the *change* of relations is potentiated, to the degree to which the individual actors cease to be the centre of attention and thinking is in terms of *coordinated relations* that permit creating viable futures through an efficacious collaboration of a communicative order. His proposal consists, basically, in the *common creation* of meaning, the co-construction of realities of relation by those involved in some problematics or others. "Communication, therefore, is seeing others confer the privilege of meaning. If others do not treat our enunciations as communication, if they do not coordinate in the proposal offered, we are reduced to the absurd".[7] Understanding itself in conversation presupposes a coordination of actions among participants through words, gaze, or corporal movements.

In consequence, the therapeutic relation entails the challenge of under-taking a collaborative journey that succeeds in dismantling and transforming the problematic matrix of the situation in an attempt to resolve, reconstruct, or dissolve it in the interest of *wellbeing*. The most important resource in the therapists' hands in this process is the *conversational act* itself and the verbal –including kinetic and proxemic – aptitudes they apply to flexibilize this relation; emphasizing in each encounter the *how*, not the *why*, of what happens. According to this focus, each movement of conversation must confer a meaning to the preceding one:

> The meaning of our words and our actions depends, from the first, on those that respond to them. And these responses lack meaning before they are, in turn, supplemented. In fact, meaning is always found in becoming, never totally consumed [but] always open to the final movement of the conversation.[8]

In any case, therapy as a relational process implies a series of theoretical movements that run from the presumed conceptual *foundations* of knowledge to the communitarian *flexibility* of meaning; from certainty to possible election; from essentialism to awareness of construction; from the professional competencies of the expert to the *democratic* collaboration of language systems; from a presumed axiological neutrality to the pondering of the values and a critical reflection on social and political aspects; from the notion of stable *mind* to that of *discourse* constructed as conversational outcome (that includes corporal and material aspects); from the unitary ego to the relational or multiple ego; from singularity to situated multivocality; from problems to possibilities; and from introspection to co-constructive action.[9]

> The general question consists in knowing whether our therapeutic practices can incite an attitude of aperture towards what is yet to come (...) Can therapy – Gergen reflects – free the participants in the conventions from static, delimited judgments, and allow them to fully cast themselves into the continual flow of relations?[10]

If therapy is conducted as a process of coordination that addresses digressions on the meaning that the event constructs and reconstructs, then this process entails the *hope* and *promise* [*sic*] that the chain of meanings will lead to the emergence of possibilities of a renewed or alternative existence that would allow the client *to live better* (according, of course, to the limits of a given point of view). In this context, the author of *Realities and Relations*[11] alludes to the so-called *poetic form* of language, by virtue of which he remits to three of its exceptional qualities: a) the capacity to question that which is common and everyday (catalysing property); b) making the imaginary believable (imaginative property); and c) provoking a sense of the aesthetic (aesthetic property). Thus, Gergen proposes the possibility of "giving life", collectively, to a *poetic dimension* in the doings of psychotherapy (which is a journey through meaning); that is, changing, more-or-less radically, the habitual dispositions of anima and action, and utilizing imagination to liberate alternative motivational sources that will be directed towards configuring more *harmonious* modes of life with the world. How is this to be achieved according to this reflection?

The first step consists in deploying a psychotherapeutic practice that "calls into question the everyday", entering into a relation that breaks away from the subject's traditional assumptions and generates a certain destabilization some definitions or perceptions or others that are entrenched in the links of that person to others. The aim is to relativize those definitions while also proposing alternative realities, other ways of *seeing* and comprehending others, opening languages that rupture the stagnation of the interpersonal world to produce a certain disequilibrium in the established modes of relation that makes it possible to re-read and re-write life histories, thus creating conversations with multiple voices. Added to this, it is necessary to foment imaginary creations in the conversation, though for Gergen this imaginative labour involves the *task* of generating discourses linked to a *positive* future; that is, a stimulating, hopeful future for the subject. In the author's words:

> The therapies that seek origins, trajectories, structures, and dynamics create the reality of the past. This reality threatens to dominate the whole conversational space of therapy. The constructionist impulse, in contrast, invites a centring on future realities, on another vision of the world, on positive perspectives, favourable results. Creating a positive vision gives direction and creates hope.[12]

Finally, Gergen proposes promoting a therapeutic link oriented towards cultivating an *aesthetic dimension* understood as "the way in which relations can give life to beauty". Of course, if in the constructionist perspective the very idea of *beauty* is a changing, cultural-linguistic construction, then the therapeutic conversation could encounter multiple elements that, in their specific context, nourish this dimension of aesthetic character. Even so, Gergen suggests using *transformational dialogues*[13] as acts of interlocution that may entail, on the one hand, the *validation* (as the instant of recognition – not refutation or annulation – of an enunciation by means of which a meaning is conferred that favours the emergence of the aesthetic); and, on the other, *dialogical metonymy* (which consists in using a fragment to express *the totality* that is desired to be manifested; and in the case of the dialogue, when the actions of an interlocutor contain *remains* or fragments of the actions of the other; that is, when interlocutors include or involve in their expressions, partially, the *presence* of the other; thus stimulating a metonymic approach). For this author, restoring that aesthetic moment in the work of psychotherapeutic intervention constitutes a "second-order challenge" that is very difficult to achieve because it must bring forth new forms of discourse, make relatively unusual conversational changes, and activate different vocabularies and/or recover the plurality of *voices*; all this as a function of weaving relations of *greater wellbeing* – less hostile or damaging – among participants.

Even though Gergen's constructionist proposal points towards promoting what he calls "a creative confluence in therapeutic practice"[14] constituted as a grand movement towards meaning (meaning shifted gradually from the *personal* to the *relational*) that also assumes consciousness of the limits of its action; even though his proposal argues for configuring an interventive practice of a reflexive, anti-essentialist and anti-authoritarian kind due to its activism in pro of a therapy without immovable foundations or transcendental arguments; even though his very reflection admits the importance of not stimulating any linguistic (or discursive) sectarian reductionism in order to recognize the existence of multiple realities (for example, body, emotions, power relations, materiality) that also participate in the construction of the meaning itself;[15] even though, in consequence, it posits the need to work "beyond the limits of spoken language" to enthusiastically vindicate the possibility of realizing inclusive connections or conjunctures (instead of exclusive disjunctures) with other combinable practices, traditionally situated and framed in different domains of activity; it is possible and necessary, in my opinion, to elaborate a critical reflection with respect to the development of Gergenian theoretics.

The key objection is, precisely, that this author *never questions the very interventive condition of psychotherapy as a practice of interlocution*. In effect, the set of proposals that he develops presuppose an acritical subsuming in the terrain of *psychological intervention* itself that is not questioned as a device of subjection or *Apparatus of the State*. As a result, his reflections on psychotherapy maintain a *pacifying* and relatively *normalizing* spirit that can function favourably for co-opting conflicts; all of which constitutes, despite its possible creative confluence and movement towards meaning, a service that supports – by flexibilizing it – the functioning of the relations of dominant knowledge and power; relations that are transformed in diverse ways to ensure their perpetuation and efficiency. In other words, when using dialogue and conversation is proposed as *resources* of intervention (both psychotherapeutic and psychosocial) to achieve the goals of wellbeing and positive coexistence in interpersonal relations, the entire project becomes another tool of the tangled institutional complex that configures that grand repair workshop of capitalism. The goal, in one way or another, is to *soften* the entrenchment of the relations of *control* characteristic of capitalist production in the contemporary world, relations that are not questioned as long as no precise, convincing impugnation of the extended ambit of *interventive praxis itself*, in all its theoretical and operative diversity, is elaborated.

Gergen's psychotherapeutic proposal does not make an evaluative review of the notion of *dialogue* itself as a cultural and political figure of current life. In fact, quite to the contrary, it unfurls a kind of *a priori* apology of that notion (and of *conversation*) through assessments that take for granted a presumed *benignity* of dialogue; thus vindicating – though with insufficient critical detainment – the epistemological and ethical utilities of dialogue applied to psychotherapy or any other social activity. But it is precisely in this cult to creative operation in hopes of *administering* human relations through the strategic figures of readaptation, of the efficacious development or transformation of people in relation to their changing environments, that the *poetic* is subordinated to the efficient mandate of the *practical* (the poetic is immersed in the *interventive mission* to be fulfilled), with which the poetic loses, indefectibly, its living nucleus before breaking out in all its rebelliousness or capacity for insurrection, in the face of the normalizing onslaughts of knowledge-power. When the poetic impulse is subjected to the lines of any interventive project (when used, for example, to *smooth things over*), it becomes a *poetic cadaver*, one that can only be stillborn in the technical territory of the timely administration and unerring diligence for reproduction and social stability.

Gilles Deleuze and Félix Guattari propose a crucial distinction of the forms of political organization based on two non-symmetrical models that, however, conserve profound mutual relations: the *Apparatuses of State* and the *Machines of war*. In this sense – Jaime Vieyra writes –

> the Apparatuses of State always seek to appropriate the Machines of war, embed them, and transform them into one more device of domination (...); while the Machines of war, for their part, by affirming their exteriority, tend to destroy the Apparatuses of State, to undo their bonds and rupture their pacts.

But the Machines of war do not have as their objective war *per se* but, rather, "a different way of occupying space (another relation with the land and beings)", of organizing human beings and "developing their affects". War becomes a complementary object when the Machinery of war creates a distinct way of living that resists the regulations and prescriptions of the Apparatuses of State, whose mission includes living *without alarms*. In this case, Gergen's poetics acts as an Apparatus of State, not as Machinery of war; that is to say, poetics as subversion, as *Machinery of war*,[16] necessarily escapes, at a certain moment, from the social devices of profitability and capture.

The schism of schizoanalysis

In contrast, and from a quite different perspective, schizoanalysis escapes from any notion of *totality* or totalizing propensity by positing the possibility of producing subjectivity in a fragmentary way in terms of differential relations of irreducible character. The aim is to account for *desiring production* itself as pure multiplicity that cannot be circumscribed to any type of unity.[17] Thus, the exercise of schizoanalysis involves a fundamental gesture of de-subjection and changing interconnection in the way of conceiving subjective experience itself and relations with the world. In this regard, Alfonso Lans observes:

> The proposal of schizoanalysis did not emerge from the nothing, it is intimately linked to some philosophies of becoming, minoritarian, revulsive, and revolutionary in nature, that find in Nietzsche their most genial exponent. He and Kierkegaard – though in clearly-differentiated directions – oppose the Kantian system, especially, the Hegelian version. Their coincidence resides in opposing repetition to all possible forms of generality.[18]

The schizoanalytic operation goes against the transcendentalist assumptions of a philosophical, theoretical, or political order to the extent that they omit the doings of contingency, randomness, *and desire itself as creative de-structuring production and as affirmative process*. It assumes a questioning that vindicates the presence of *becoming* as a key condition for the re-appropriation of a thinking that flees from the orderings, hierarchies, and categorizations of science (of positivist spirit) in the analysis of the complex productions of subjectivity in the context of capitalism. It constitutes, in effect, a historical-social conception of contemporary subjective productions. It criticizes the idea of the stable and the permanent in all scientific-social conceptions that de-personalize thinking and separate it from a corporal and material dimension that supports its conjugations. It impugns modern thinking, the ascetism of pretended objectivity in social reflection and, provokingly, inconveniently, and irreverently, makes an epistemological and political critique of a *transdisciplinary* character of the totalizing condition of many established theoretical apparatuses in the study of subjectivity, the unconscious, and culture, especially orthodox psychoanalysis.

Schizoanalysis proposes composing the ethical-aesthetic dimensions "that directly signal the political as constitutive of the practice of analysis and, therefore, as the diagrammer of the Unconscious".[19] With respect to *intervention*, schizoanalysis resists the extended professionalisms and corporativisms of the institutionalized practices of the *psychological complex*, holding that any schizoanalytic intervention or *task* will be linked to inciting intensive, interconnected processes of desiring production that participate in the open, creative recomposition of the concrete world in which we live. It speaks of promoting *molecular* – singular, minimal, micropolitical – revolutions against *molar* – majoritarian, massive, global – orderings and, with this, of inventing alternative existential plexuses. In this way, schizoanalysis breaks away from disciplinary controls and the apparatuses of social regulation (including the psychological complex) expressed even in the *humanist* project that tends towards a vision of the subject as functionality and full personal "realization", in the end, at the service of the capitalist system. In its anti-conservatism, schizoanalysis opens the possibility of transiting multiple lines of escape and subversion that vindicate madness and desire against the established institutional designs of sanity and normality. Schizoanalysts, therefore, must separate themselves from "all hegemonic or prophetic pretension" and procure the constant mutation of a molar perspective of the world as integration to an unfinished molecular interconnection of diverse relations that inaugurate alternative (divergent, unusual) forms of social and personal life. Alfonso Lans comments:

In reality, the scientific ideal is embodied as a policy to develop, not only as foundation of the politics of State, but by directly producing a technocratic power that penetrates and reconstructs the social tissue by codifying it (over-codification). This operation of generalized statification is made viable through such ideological apparatuses as the judiciary, education, hygiene, the police, semiotics, linguistic [systems], etc. that, moreover, tend to become globalized. Thus, we see how an army of techniques of diverse disciplines laminates the social such that conflicts abandon the 'battlefields' and pass to fill the cabinets of distinct professionals (*experts*) whose function is to re-diagram the social. It is in this atmosphere that we must understand how professionals and intellectuals are aligned today.[20]

This is why schizoanalysis does not seek to design – for example – policies to promote health or "prevent" social problems that support and justify interventive practices to ensure the reproductive functioning and normalization of behaviours and values in the population. Rather, schizoanalysis is oriented towards rethinking subjective and existential production in terms of constant material and axiological revolution. It is oriented towards generating spaces for the journey of those molecular and micro-political lines of reinvention of the social world itself.

In this sense, the tasks that schizoanalysis proposes act as an antidote so that this is not confused with a new disciplinary device, however special it may be, for its destructive tasks signal that it cannot cease to affect itself so as to never stop making everything begin again.[21]

In effect, in the face of the exercise of *ontological and political capture* presupposed and developed by the diverse forms of psychological intervention in modernity, schizoanalysis sets out to prevent the corresponding institutions from installing and imposing – unopposed – the criteria of a functional, efficient life in accordance with the current demands of capitalism. It opposes the pretension of the theoretical-technical devices of the psychological complex to *unify* the world and collective life, people, and things in the values and prescriptions of a bourgeois *familiarism* (that ignores, disowns, or denies the very social and diverse character of existence) and to reduce the notion of madness to the psychiatric taxonomies of the technocracy. For this reason, schizoanalysis tends to undo the devices of institutional action that conceive and deal with *mental illness* as an object of research and professional work.

All production of subjectivity and all affective load (cathexis) remit in their flows to diverse, broad historical-social fields that are superimposed and amply surpass the specific field of the family and its concrete relations. In any case, capitalist society promotes the *schizophrenising sinking* from its very structure, as a means of production that involves precise economic and political circuits. The social field is not reduced to its familiar expression or translation but, rather, entails complex connections and desiring loads of all kinds. This explains why the schizoanalytic reflection cannot aspire to constitute just one more disciplinary system of intervention, or a professional specialization of psychiatric, psychoanalytical, or psychosocial character. Nor does it have an *omnicomprehensive* intention, but constitutes only sets of practices and inventions (produced concomitantly – or laterally – to established disciplinary procedures) that strive to connect, reconnect, and interconnect lines of molecular escape to reactivate desiring production and existential de-subjection.

The schizoanalyst, then, is not defined as a scenic director for the *theatre* of life, but as an artisan or, perhaps better, a mechanic that works with *desiring machines* (in effect, since a key aspect of schizoanalysis is the notion of *production*, it articulates the positing of desiring machines as elements of an intensive and specific or singular nature supported by multiplicities whose interpenetration and combinations give rise to – that is, produce – all that which constitutes reality itself).

Schizoanalytic work, therefore, remits to a heterogeneity that includes the linguistic sphere but is not reduced to it. It involves the group as disposition and concrete psychosocial networks in the machination of the subject himself, while questioning the presumed totality (insuperable or absolute character) of the utilities of language. In *groupality*, ecological, economic, aesthetic, corporal, or ethological aspects come to be articulated in different ways that cannot be subsumed in any semiology of language. For this reason, schizoanalysis is separate from a structuralist vision of speech that denies or eludes the problem of the immanent production of subjectivity as emotional, aesthetic, and micro-political rupture with respect to the discursive-dominant vectors instituted in society.

By opposing all closed conceptualization or structuration that acts as a way to capture or freeze becoming, schizoanalysis assumes that the real is given in that immanent and open movement that cannot be petrified by the immobile cut of the transcendent *concept*. Moreover, as Nicolás Bourriaud reiterates, in the schizoanalytic proposal:

... aesthetics enjoys a status apart. It constitutes a 'paradigm', a flexible device capable of functioning on different levels, on different planes of knowing. First, as the base that allows it to articulate its 'ecosophy'; as a model of production of subjectivity; as an instrument to fecundate psychiatric-psychoanalytical practice (...). It appeals to aesthetics to counteract the hegemony of the 'superego advocate of scientificism' that stereotypes analytical practices in formulas that (in this case Guattari) reproach the 'psy community'; it is returning to the past, manipulating Freudian or Lacanian concepts as if they were insuperable truths (...). According to Guattari, the aesthetic paradigm is called to contaminate all records of discourse, to inoculate the poison of creative uncertainty and delirious invention in all fields of knowledge.[22]

In any case, schizoanalysis vindicates the intensive time of *event*, of the productive becoming of creation. In this sense, we are dealing with a *poetic* movement. Contrary to the exercise of constructing, configuring, presenting, verbalizing, comprehending, interpreting (and, of course, analysing) the familiar *novel* of the subject that becomes patent – in, for example, orthodox psychoanalysis and many forms of psychotherapy – with the explicit or implicit questions "what has happened?", "what is about to happen?", schizoanalysis recovers the *poetic* moment as a mutant, cinematographic, unusual, aporetic, and somehow delirious, invention in the search for de-subjection. More than *novelising*, it is *poeticising*, imagining, the production of desire as creative force. But this requires, above all, the capacity to detach from any theoretical conception or pre-determining reading apparatus of perception that operates under the sponsorship of dominant knowledge-power at that moment. This means – as Alfonso Lans ironizes – "that at the first Mama-Papa we do not shout out Oedipus, Oedipus! – that is, the magic formula – because the problem may be oedipal or some other, or may be overflowing".[23]

The technical-conceptual apparatuses of psychological reading and intervention are deployed with a willingness to crush the *desiring machines*. It is necessary to avoid not only the aprioristic reduction of the field to be traversed, but also imaginative sterility, precipitated by the censure that tends to be imposed on the possibility of inventing alternate worlds. For this same reason, schizoanalysis is not circumscribed to the spoken or written word, but remits to complex networks of objects in the material world and to artistic-intellectual-subjective practices and products of varied sign. It recovers the singularization of thought, of feeling, of saying, and of doing as the subversive banner it raises against the generalizations and technical-methodological efficiencies of the different modalities of intervention in the psychological complex. It generates other perspectives and modes of interaction for the interweaving of new existential plexuses, *playing inventively*, somehow fleeing from existing rules and prescriptions; escaping from established representations; venturing out: following events, navigating without instruments and acceding, precisely, to *meaning*; even though there is no event or meaning that is not linked to some multiplicity or other. Schizoanalysis tends towards the *active utopia*; the act of freedom that regenerates subjective life in terms of unrepeatable (*artistic*) singularity.

It is possible to think of a *desiring dialogue* produced through non-centralist links and points of dispersion by virtue of which a kind of time made of existential fragments in relation is inaugurated. Such a dialogue does not represent anything; nor does it pretend to achieve certain tacit or explicit objectives; and it cannot be prescribed institutionally. In schizoanalytic terms, this dialogue might be thought as a possible instance of the articulation and emergence of desiring machines, continually in a state of suspense due to the simultaneous presence of molar machines that seek efficiency. But, in any case, it does not dialogue with people as much as with vast, complex, changing *worlds*. It is less a *human* dialogue (let's say, strictly interpersonal), than a *not purely human* dialogue; that is, one interconnected with molecular mechanistic elements of unpredictable singularity. Psychopoetic dialogue is, then, less *anthropomorphic* than the interventive dialogue that operates through in-formative prescription. That dialogue of intervention entails (by *law*) an anthropomorphic molar configuration of interlocution directed implacably towards one *transcendence* or another. In opposition to this design, desiring dialogue ignores prescriptions as often as it can; it does not seek transcendence because it constitutes (in its fleeting act) an instant of energetic and productive positivity sustained by multiplicities of de-subjection, creative transcodification, and *nomadic conjunctions*.

The dialogue of psychological intervention constitutes a *theatre*, a *scenario* where meaningful dramatic roles assigned previously by the theatre *company* are presented. Psychopoetic dialogue, in contrast, constitutes an open *factory*, one that is mutant, a traveller of new subjective meanings; a factory whose key characteristic resides in its distancing from all things *axiomatic*. If interventive dialogue culminates in an adaptive neo-idealness or neo-suitability that is more-or-less functional for the participating subject or subjects, psychopoetic, or desiring dialogue claims in every moment its immanent materiality and its useless, inconclusive character. Unlike the organizational, structural installation of interventive dialogue, *psychopoetic* dialogue produces words and desiring bodies in a disorganized way in an intense, varied link that opens infinite possibilities, beyond *linguistic chess*, towards a kind of *game of bingo* where

> now a word, now a drawing, now a thing or a fragment of something emerges, depending one upon others, only by the order of aleatory sorting, remaining together due only to the absence of bonds (non-localizable bonds), without possessing any more status than being dispersed elements of desiring machines that are also dispersed.[24]

This is why if psychological intervention in its different modalities promotes dialogues that *reterritorialize* diverse representations and beliefs in the subject (towards the reconstruction of molar complexes), the desiring dialogue of psychopoetics suddenly intrudes as a machine of existential and intersubjective *deterritorialization* that inaugurates factories of errant affectivity, even though this deterritorialization of the flows of desire occurs in union (simultaneously) with other possible reterritorializations of greater or lesser coverage and permanence. But if psychological intervention, by means of the dialogical devices it implants, forms part of that grand *social axiomatics* that operates as a function of consolidating the system according to the requirements of the market and in accordance with the need to promote the acquisition and application of verbal, technical, or emotional *competencies* in order to achieve efficiency in some reproductive activities or others in today's globalized world, then it is necessary to *resist*: to reinvent the notion and life of *dialogue* in the discovery of an interlocution that emerges as a desiring machine: a discourse that declassifies; that advances along a *crazy vector*[25]; that moves counter to all interventive vocation; that plays subversively in its heterogeneous recreation of the world; that produces subjectivity and that claims in multiple ways, the poetic instance as fleeting, unpredictable, and uncontrolled event.[26]

Notes

1 Jodorowsky, A. (2004) *Psicomagia*. Mexico: Grijalbo.
2 See for example: Herrera, R. (2008) *Poética del psicoanálisis*. Mexico: Siglo XXI.
3 Gergen, K. (2006) *Construir la realidad. El futuro de la psicoterapia*. Barcelona: Paidós, pp. 173–184.
4 Elkaïm, M. Prefacio. In: Gergen, K. (2006) *Construir la realidad. El futuro de la psicoterapia*. Ed. cit. pp. 12–13.

5 Gergen, K. (n3) p. 33. These reflections maintain clear affinities with J. Shotter's proposal (2001) *Realidades conversacionales. La construcción de la vida a través del lenguaje.* Buenos Aires: Amorrortu.

6 Idem, pp. 38–39.

7 Idem, p. 66.

8 Idem, p. 81.

9 Idem, pp. 87–115.

10 Idem, p. 133.

11 Gergen, K. (1996) *Realidades y relaciones. Aproximaciones a la construcción social.* Barcelona: Paidós.

12 Gergen, K. *Construir la realidad.* Ed. cit. p. 181.

13 See: Gergen, K.; McNamee, S.; Barret, F. (2002) Realizing transformative dialogue. In: Roberts, N.C. (Comp.) *The Transformative Power of Dialogue.* New York: Elsevier Science, pp. 77–105.

14 Gergen, K. *Construir la realidad.* Ed. cit. pp. 193–206.

15 Idem, pp. 197–199.

16 See: Vieyra, J. (1999) Deleuze y la máquina de guerra zapatista. *Utopía 1,* 9–12, and, of course, Deleuze, G.; Guattari, F. (1980) *Mil mesetas. Capitalismo y esquizofrenia.* Valencia: Pretextos, 2002, especially section 12: "1227 – Tratado de nomadología: La máquina de guerra" pp. 359–431.

17 Deleuze, G.; Guattari, F. (1972) *El Anti-Edipo. Capitalismo y esquizofrenia.* Barcelona: Paidós, 1998, pp. 283–392.

18 Lans, A. (2005) Esquizoanálisis. In: Romero, J.; Álvaro, R. (Eds.) (2005) *Psicópolis. Paradigmas actuales y alternativos en la psicología contemporánea.* Barcelona: Kairós, pp. 313–361, p. 324. For an introductory review of schizoanalytic proposals, see the excellent text by Gregorio Baremblitt (2004) on schizoanalysis in *Subjetividad y Cultura 21,* 29–41. By the same author: (1998) *Introduçâo a esquizoanálise.* Belo Horizonte: Biblioteca do Instituto Felix Guattari.

19 Idem, p. 336.

20 Idem, pp. 337–338.

21 Idem, p. 339.

22 Bourriaud, N. (2006) *Estética relacional.* Buenos Aires: Adriana Hidalgo, pp. 120–121. In the final chapter, "Hacia una política de las formas", the author addresses the problem of limits, status, and the functioning of individual subjectivity and art in relation to the work of Deleuze and (above all) Guattari (pp. 99–131). Another important evaluation of Guattari's thought is in González, F. (2002) *Sujeto y subjetividad. Una aproximación histórico-cultural.* Mexico: Thompson, pp. 98–105.

23 Lans, A. (n18) p. 349.

24 Idem, p. 319. See also, the beautiful text on the intensification of randomness or the infusion of chaos in the cosmos, "La lotería en Babilonia" by J.L. Borges (1944) *Ficciones.* Buenos Aires: Sur.

25 Deleuze, G.; Guattari, F. (n17) p. 406.

26 I am forever grateful for the academic labours of Dr. Daniel Tarnovsky (University of Buenos Aires), whose writings and conferences stimulated my interest in schizoanalytic thought. See for example: Tarnovsky, D. (2001) *Globalización, síntoma y angustia. Crisis planetaria y subjetividad.* Conference presented in the Universidad Iberoamericana, Mexico City, October, 2001.

PART II
The event of psychopoetics

4

LANGUAGE: ORDER-WORD AND MINORITARIAN BECOMING

When some people speak with others they produce not only a certain transmission of information, but also establish diverse forms of relation, generating behavioural effects or achieving a more-or-less predefined objective. Speaking, therefore, constitutes one of the most immediate expressions of the ongoing transformation of the subject: when one speaks, one becomes other things (the one becomes many). However, all speech also entails or presupposes links; in reality, it realizes and actualizes some process of enunciation. In the view of Deleuze and Guattari, in fact, acts of enunciation and the enunciate itself, as a fundamental linguistic unity, are associated with the notion of *order-word*. Language must in some way be related to the milieu of *obedience*. "A grammatical rule – they point out – [is] more fundamentally a marker of power than a syntactic marker". This situation spans the entire communicative exercise: "Information is only the strict minimum necessary for the emission, transmission, and observation of orders as commands".[1] Language gives orders to life. In their everyday movement and realization, order-words entail something akin to a *verdict*, a kind of *death sentence*. In this sense, it is necessary to understand that *dialoguing* – as verbalized language – is an exercise that does not remit to *neutral* codes, nor can it be reduced to mere communication of information. In the emergence of dialogue there exists an inescapable *pragmatic* and *political* dimension that turns out to be at least as important as the semantic or syntactic field. Therefore, the specific meanings produced in the dialogue are defined, as well, by the acts that

DOI: 10.4324/9781003129295-4

the enunciation presupposes at each instant. But the enunciation – we must keep in mind – endures the order-word.

> We call order-words, not a particular category of explicit statements (for example, in the imperative), but the relation of every word or every statement to implicit presuppositions, in other words, to speech acts that are, and can only be, accomplished in the statement. Order-words do not concern commands only, but every act that is linked to statements by a "social obligation." Every statement displays this link, directly or indirectly. Questions, promises, are order-words. The only possible definition of language is the set of all order-words, implicit presuppositions, or speech acts current in a language at a given moment.[2]

More than informing or communicating, language transmits order-words in the vertebration of social mandates; that is, in the realization of life. The linkage between act and enunciate ensures the advance of the order-word. However, it will also be possible to promote a certain *linguistic indiscipline* as an exercise of opposition to the structuring *discipline* of the enunciation and *grammaticality* (which defines the *correct* use of language through precepts). But, clearly, this presupposes that the realization of a dialogical encounter will not produce any meaning absolutely independent of the significations traced by the enunciative-grammatical (and practical-political) *doctrine* that is dominant in that moment, or in a specific social field. The processes of subjectivation will unfailingly be related to the corresponding orders of subjection. In fact, order-words, in their enormous variability, possess the capacity to make themselves forgotten by speakers. No one is to blame for the order-words that she/he has followed and transmitted in interaction and conversations throughout their lifetime. Order-words have, hence, the will of *indirect* discourse and, in many cases, of silent realization.

Each individual enunciation current in the dialogue constitutes, in some way, the resonance of those collective and impersonal *mandates*. The production of subjectivity is, in a certain way, a *relative process* that bonds to the requirements of the discursive axes extended by sociality. The enunciative moment is not, however, exhausted by the confirmation of *constants* of the discourse (that is, by the acceptance and recognition of, and subordination to, the established courses of reality), for it also entails, as an element inaccessible to normative determinations, the emergence of the *transformation* of the world itself, an act that upon being performed constitutes what is "expressed" by the enunciate. Here, we are dealing with those instantaneous acts by virtue of which, for example, the accused is converted into the condemned by what the judge pronounces in her/his sentence; the youngster reaches the age of majority by that which is stipulated in a specific regulation of civil character; or the passengers on a hijacked airplane are transformed into hostages by the declarations of the hijackers.

This leads Deleuze and Guattari to speak of *incorporeal transformations*, alluding to the *acts of transformation of realities* that, though attributed to the diverse *bodies* that experience those changes directly ("bodies" understood in the broad sense, not only as anatomic-physiological bodies, but as *social* bodies, like juridical, moral, and psychological apparatuses, etc.). These occur, rather, as attributes that are not corporeal because they are, precisely, *what is expressed* by the enunciate in relation to such social bodies.

> … incorporeal transformation is recognizable by its instantaneousness, its immediacy, by the simultaneity of the statement expressing the transformation and the effect the transformation produces (…) Love is an intermingling of bodies that can be represented by a heart with an arrow through it, by a union of souls, etc., but the declaration "I love you" expresses a noncorporeal attribute of bodies, the lover's as well as that of the loved one.[3]

The transformation of such realities is said of the bodies involved, but the *transformation* is, in itself, *incorporeal* and remits to the corresponding enunciation. In this way, *corporeal modifications* are distinguished from *incorporeal transformations*: two different formulas, one of *content*, the other of *expression*. Thus, *expression* will be constituted by the concatenation of "the expressed" – that is, by the chaining of the different elements of the expressed – while *content* will be constituted by "the actions and passions of bodies"; for example: "When knife cuts flesh, when food or poison spreads through the body, when a drop of wine falls into water, there is an intermingling of bodies; but the statements, "The knife is cutting the flesh", "I am eating", "The water is turning red", express incorporeal transformations of an entirely different nature (…)".[4] What these incorporeal transformations reveal is, precisely, the notion of *event*.

The event is a value that is not corporeal but one that, while attributed to bodies, is not reduced to the corporeal condition with which the body is related. The event is not the representation of a content, it is not explained directly by the corporeal plot in itself, nor by the play of references. The event may well imply, at some moment, an *act of language*. An enunciate speaks not of the *things per se*, but of the *states of things and from the proper states of things.* Between content and expression there will be a relatively independent functioning and, at the same time, a certain reciprocal presupposition that impedes proposing a primordial character to one or the other.

Moreover, both content and expression (which live in constant interaction) inescapably imply through their conjugations, an intense, movement away from permanent *deterritorialization.* Content does not determine expression through causal action, but this does not mean that expression constitutes a self-sufficient form understood as a linguistic system that makes it possible to erect an *abstract language machine* of a linear character; that is, one that considers the linguistic elements as *constant per se.* The act of the enunciation is not merely linguistic, but also *diagrammatic* and *over-linear,* in effect, in opposition to a fixed linear linguistic order (that only *reproduces* reality) what appear are the very incorporeal transformations or *events* that already involve a certain over-linearity because they imply, precisely, an interpenetration between language and the related social and political fields with which reality itself is transformed. The linguistic is part of the complex diagram of the enunciation, not the opposite, so, it is pertinent to speak of innumerable symbioses and mixtures that occur in the enunciation (saying "stirrup" – for example – presupposes a new and interesting "man-horse" relation with all the instrumental derivations at its core).

Is not, therefore, possible to accept the existence of constant universals of language that permit perceiving it strictly as a homogeneous system for the reproduction of the established orders of reality. In truth, variation is inherent to all systems and operates from within. All *systems* change, jump, flee from themselves, for they all include a potential for acting transformation. This occurs to such a degree that all systems can be defined not so much by their constants (which tend towards transcendent homogeneity), but by their *variability* (which presupposes immanence and continuity, though they are objects of specific regulations). This continuous variation of language, which involves an ongoing variation of reality in itself, occurs in the everyday enunciations of people: "In the course of a single day, an individual repeatedly passes from language to language. He successively speaks as "father to son" and as a boss; to his lover, he speaks an infantilized language; while sleeping he is plunged into an oniric discourse, then abruptly returns to a professional language when the telephone rings".[5] These are not extrinsic variations but intrinsic ones. When one speaks as *father, husband,* or *professional,* one manifests internal changes of a syntactic, semantic and, of course, phonological, and prosodic order. But one also, and simultaneously, manifests changes of an existential order. Language, therefore, like the world, lives crisscrossed intrinsically by vectors of continuous variation.

In the face of the *centralizing* function of discursive constants (that mark the establishment and entrenchment of the orders of reality) what emerges is the decentring instant of continuous variations upon speaking. While some centres of *validity* and *stability* or other function when speaking, supported by the designation of the extended social apparatuses of knowledge and power, such *establishments* of the enunciation organize the *major modes* of the realization of speech itself and of the world; it also happens that a potency is effectuated, one that is resistant to those central zones, while some *minor modes* or others occur (fleetingly) by virtue of which there comes a resurgence of the infinity of alternative elements that tend to disperse the unicity of that which is said and of that which is. Phantasmagorical, imaginary, idiosyncratic elements habitually charged with unusual emotional chromatisms that somehow *decompose* the central principle of the enunciation to promote incessant forms of change in the meanings involved at the moment they are expressed. This variation thus frees itself such that its realization weaves the threads of creativity.

In this sense, the so-called secret languages, like *argot* or professional *jargon*, and the special languages used by sentinels and salespeople, invent their own lexicons and rhetorical forms that differ from the aspects normally manifested by language in common use. This confirms the existence of ongoing variations of the dominant language-world-system; enunciative manifestations that, while they may be seen as *sub-systems* of hierarchical centres, disrupt those linguistic territories generalized by sociality. It is a type of *chromatic* speech that implies an enormous *coefficient of variation*. While this also entails installing certain fixations or operative constants, these in no way maintain a *definitive* condition. If the linguistic system tends to remain in the major modes of the enunciation – that is, in the cultivation of the dominant, universal constancy, and transcendence – then all language in its concrete realization also tends towards immanent, unpredictable, intense, innovative variation.

One thing that may occur during dialogue or conversation is that one language may be created or exercised *inside* another; an enunciative *sub-system* that is more-or-less spurious, apocryphal, or *nomadic*, may be dynamized with respect to the discursive patterns installed by the axes of constancy of the dominant language-world-system (axes of constancy that extend, of course, with the vocation of perpetuity). This situation reveals a certain *bilingualism* of dialogue and conversation, even when this occurs in the same language. In other words, any person who dialogues, who speaks with another, always does so by putting into play *two languages*: the language of the order-word and that of obedience (that is, the language of the establishment and functional reproduction of the reality just as it is), and the language of variation and creativity (that is, the language of the disobedient transformation of the world). Each speaker, in his/her expressions, gestures, and words, thus produces unrepeatable *methods* of variation: opening the heterogeneous spectrum of enunciative possibilities to alter, in this way, the diachronic deployment of *sedentary* language (entrusted with installing, validating, and permanently fixing the reality made available by dominant knowledge and power).

The language in use always involves unrealized potentialities. The constant determinations of standard speech and of the functional realization of the world – for example, in the exercise of dialogue – suffer the *assault* of unpredictable variation, variation that promotes atypical turns in the expression that on many occasions turn out to be impertinent. As verbal act, it modifies *correct* forms of speech, thereby questioning its prescriptive constancy. What is produced, then, is a tension that *deterritorialises* the dominant language-world-system. Thus it is that unusual expression generates intensive reliefs in verbal exchanges and opens unexpected alternatives of communicative follow-up. It is interesting that atypical expression (surprising, unusual, inventive) is not subject, obviously, to the correct (constant, reiterative) forms of speech, but that it cannot constitute an absolute variable. Unusual expression eliminates the *specific weight* from the constant because it utilizes that constant in a different way, one that is inadequate, disobedient, or incorrect with respect to the generalized routes of its application in the extended speech of the collectivity. Moreover, it adds a certain, characteristic, emotional colour that alters the grey tones of enunciative discipline.

These variations do not have to be seen as isolated phenomena or exclusive to *children*, *madmen*, or *poets*. Variations embody the ordinary doings of language. Variations are not marginal because language – I insist – does not have to be defined only by *constants*, does not have to be conceived as *universal* or *general instance*, for it can also be perceived as *potential-real instance* that does not admit obligatory, absolute, definitive, or invariable rules. What language contains are only "optional rules that ceaselessly vary with variation itself, as in a game in which each move changes the rules".[6]

Deleuze and Guattari elaborated a critique of the linguistic postulate which holds that language can only be studied *scientifically* under the conditions of a standard-major-language-system. A scientific study of language should strive to extract variables from a set of constants in order to determine the series of constant relations among those variables.

But the scientific model taking language as an object of study is one with the political model by which language is homogenized, centralized, standardized, becoming a language of power, a major or dominant language. Linguistics can claim all it wants to be science, nothing but pure science – it wouldn't be the first time that the order of pure science was used to secure the requirements of another order.[7]

Any sign, including grammaticality, will be a marker of power before being a syntactic marker. The capacity of the *normal* subject to produce grammatically adequate, correct phrases and expressions constitutes a condition of possibility that is basic for their own subjection to the laws and regulations of social life (this is inevitable as all people learn to speak, in principle, in order to be subjected). When someone ignores the dominant grammaticality and begins to express her/himself in a distinct manner – for example, *incoherently* or designating the world with neologisms – she or he will very likely find themselves shut away in a psychiatric hospital or some other *special* institution. The unity of a language has, therefore, a character both ontological and political. It is in this way that the efforts of science to delimit the constants, regularities, and/or stable relations in the study of its object, go hand-in-hand with political strivings – often ignored – that seek to impose such aspects on everyday praxis (in this case, on speech); that is, of promoting *order-words*.

According to these authors it is possible, nonetheless, to differentiate between two types of language, *high* and *low* or, perhaps better, *major* and *minor*, though in reality these refer less to two types of languages than to two possible ways of *treating* the same language. The first treatment is defined by the power of the constants, the second by the potency of variation. What happens is that no homogeneous system can exist that is not linked to immanent, continuous, *minoritarian* variations through which the system continues to constitute itself.

Dialoguing and conversing can lead to a *minor* becoming of the *major* language. It is possible to achieve a *deterritorialisation* of the traditional mandates of a certain dialogical or conversational reason installed at a given moment; transform the *major* dialogical praxis into the *minor one*; flee from conclusive, closed, let's say, fully realized dialogue; dialogue and converse in one's own language, but in unison; activate a foreignizing point in speech; follow the *majoritarian* mandates of that dialogue (this is inescapable), but also open *minor worlds* that fragment the *major* dialogical installation in unpredictable ways. It is, then, to the degree to which someone traces minor lines of aperture or digression (speculative, parodic, burlesque, imaginative, metaphoric) in the context of the realization of a major dialogical reason (epistemological, algorithmic, institutional) that the event of *psychopoetics* manifests itself in its evanescence and in its elusive character (in the form of an incorporeal transformation).

Psychopoetics is related to the possibility of achieving a kind of – partial – foreignizing of the dialogical encounter. At that instant, one renounces the pretension of full analytical understanding. It is no longer so important *what* is said, or *who* says it, but the creative vertebration of the existential plexuses involved in this interlocution that becomes *minoritarian*.

We must recall that the "majoritarian" and "minoritarian" constitute two functional dimensions of the use of language, not just a quantitative opposition.

> Majority implies a constant, of expression or content, serving as a standard measure by which to evaluate it. Let us suppose that the constant or standard is the average adult-white-heterosexual-European-male-speaking a standard language (…). It is obvious that "man" holds the majority, even if he is less numerous than mosquitoes, children, women, blacks, peasants, homosexuals (…). Majority assumes a state of power and domination, not the other way around. It assumes the standard measure, not the other way around.[8]

In this sense, all determination distinct from the constant sustains a *minoritarian* condition. This means that it will have the status of *sub-system*, or will perform a movement that tends towards *exiting* the system, towards existence as an *outsider*. In addition, however, the *majority*, by virtue of enjoying the support of the dominant standard measure of which it is made up, never loses its protagonism, always promises to achieve *success* ("you can only come to be *someone* in life if you follow the rules"). The *minority*, in contrast, never attains *success*, has no protagonists, and tends to be associated with the *nobody* but, for this very reason, "is the becoming of everybody, one's potential becoming to the extent that one deviates from the model".[9]

The *majoritarian* then, constitutes the homogeneous, constant system; the minorities constitute sub-systems; and the *minoritarian* constitutes the potential becoming – created and creative – of the world. It is not a question of *conquering the majority*; that is, of converting the minoritarian into the majoritarian (by installing another *constant* that dominates from other symbolic points). What occurs is that *becoming* is never *majoritarian*;

becoming is *minoritarian becoming*, a *minor speech* in dialogue and in conversation that enables a becoming which involves, of course, the entire system; a minor speech that acts as a potential agent of change and erosion of the structure of that dialogical encounter as *majoritarian* dimension. It is about a minor becoming of the major dialogue: "Minorities (...) must also be thought of as seeds, crystals of becoming whose value is to trigger uncontrollable movements and deterritorializations of the mean or majority".[10]

The positions or formulations confronted in a dialogue (that is, that which a subject utters – her/his thesis – in counterposition to other ideas – antithesis – proposed by an interlocutor who is recognized as a dialogant) lose preponderance in themselves, because what now stands out is the whole set of emergent – not consensual – aspects that are unpredictable, de-authorized, and creative, and that constitute at that moment, the expression of the very minoritarian becoming of the exercise of dialogue as *system*. The *minoritarian conscience* is what becomes *world-creation* by dialoguing. It incorporates the continuous variation that transgresses, constantly and in different ways, the frontiers of the majoritarian standard measure of the discursive orders that fix *world-conservation*. Minoritarian conscience in dialogue thus invents specific becomings in the *conjugation* of the world.

It is in these terms that dialogue as the vehicle of order-words continues to function in discursive interaction. It is dialogue that complies with the mandates of knowledge and power that circulate in any given cultural or institutional apparatus. Here, we are dealing with that *deadly-mortifying* moment of dialogue:

> Order-words bring immediate death to those who receive the order, or potential death if they do not obey, or a death they must themselves inflict, take elsewhere. A father orders to his son, "You will do this", "You will not do that", cannot be separated from the little death sentence the son experiences on a point of his person. Death, death; it is the only judgment, and it is what makes judgment a system. The verdict.

This is why one *dies*, in a certain sense, upon receiving-obeying-reproducing the order-word in dialogue, just as when one dialogues *by order-word*. Nonetheless, the order-word carries within itself something else that is bonded to it, something like "a warning cry or a message to flee. It would be oversimplifying to say that flight is a reaction against the order-word; rather, it is included in it, as its other face in a complex assemblage, its other component".[11]

When one dialogues, converses, speaks with anyone, *order-word* and *flight* are involved. It is to these complexities that *continuous variation* obeys-responds. Continuous flight and variation intensively oppose the extensive installation (by order-word) of the mortifying discourse; in other words: the devil opposes God. Continuous variation in the realization of a dialogue would thus suppose rupturing moulds; overstepping instituted limits; fluidity of events, and with this, the impugnation of all word or body that pretends to *settle* in some clearly demarcated point. The continuous variation of content and expression that occurs when effectuating a dialogical or conversational exercise implies that the words, bodies, gestures, things, *reality* itself in all its heterogeneity, are *affected* by those who participate in that interlocution; an affectation that will descend in ways yet unknown: vibration, intermittence, chromatism, variegation, vivification, multiplicity.

The crucial question will not involve the pretension of annulling the action of the order-word (for this is impossible) but, rather, how to rebel (and reveal oneself) against the *death sentence*, against the intimate death that the order-word comes to inoculate in the blood of those who speak. The crucial question will be how to open oneself to disquietude and laughter; how to wield *competencies* for a certain provisional-tactical-strategic flight from the totalizing discursive scheme and then for the combative and ludic return, through the clout of action and unusual word against the constants of essentialism.

> There are pass-words beneath order-words. Words that pass, words that are components of passage, whereas order-words mark stoppages or organized, stratified compositions. A single thing or word undoubtedly has this twofold nature: it is necessary to extract one from the other – to transform the compositions of order into components of passage.[12]

But in any case, a dialogue or conversation whose emergence implies the modification of a certain *composition of order* in *components of passage*, is a dialogue that, fortunately, is *decomposed* creatively in the very act of its realization; it is a conversational encounter that breaches the mandates of knowledge and of power; a dialogue that becomes minoritarian; that is, a speech that allows itself to be carried away – *psychopoetically* – by the improvised music of the *event*.

Notes

1 Deleuze, G.; Guattari, F. (1987) *A Thousand Plateaus. Capitalism and Schizophrenia*. Minneapolis: University of Minnesota Press, p. 76.
2 Idem, p. 79.
3 Idem, p. 81.
4 Idem, p. 86.
5 Idem, p. 94.
6 Idem, p. 100.
7 Idem, p. 101.
8 Idem, p. 105.
9 Idem, p. 105.
10 Idem, p. 106.
11 Idem, p. 107.
12 Idem, p. 110.

5

INTUITIVE PLOT, AFFECTIVE REASON, AND INSTANT THOUGHT

The western worlds of so-called *postmodernity* today participate in diverse social practices with the return of a series of *archaic values* placed on a first plane of interactive life. Accompanying the weakening of certainties in thought, juvenile phenomena like new *tribalisms* and *nomadisms* emerge that entails as well, in the strict sense, a *tragic* attitude towards life revealed in multiple episodes of everyday experience; social practices that in the absence of that referent, seem to make no sense. Through this *tragic sensitivity* postmodern time seems to stop: to live a kind of immobilization or, at least, to become slower in contrast to the accelerated scientific, technological, and economic development of modernity with its eminently *dramatic* sign. For the sociologist Michel Maffesoli, social life today seems, rather, to be a concatenation of *frozen instants* that seem to be the basis for the key imperative of *re-creation*. This is a paradigm change that runs from an *ego-centred* conception of the world – that grants primacy to the rational individual living in the contractual society of modernity – to a *locus-centred* conception related to the emergence of the groups or *neo-tribes* of contemporary social life that, in turn, generate specific spaces of coexistence in the nascent postmodernity.[1]

Modern individualism is, then, dramatic, while postmodern tribal activity is tragic. In that tragic condition Maffesoli includes moments of unbridled jubilation, of effervescence for life. The notion of *history,* as a central category of the analysis of modernity, is relativized. We pass from a singular, linear time founded upon the idea of project, to another time, this one cyclic, recursive, *presentist* that seeks to disassociate itself from

DOI: 10.4324/9781003129295-5

bourgeois utilitarianism, and bears the sign of plurality. We are attending a certain reactivation of *archaic* values, and ways of being and thinking that since the epoch of *enlightened* modernity had remained in the domain of a presumed *obscurantism*.

Modes of life that are less rational and more *Dionysian*; less sedentary and more *nomadic*, that involve, in one way or another, many contemporary practices. We are dealing with a *vitalism* that invites the scandalous laughter of new paganisms in the face of the aging of the worlds of seriousness and disciplined programming, the rebirth of a polysemic vitality that does not follow the steps of that innocent and optimistic progressivism of other times, thus living a logic of conjunction more than of disjunction with the emergence of attitudes of *immediacy* in the new generations, oriented towards diverse neo-tribal hedonisms and mimetics in a framework of permanent reversibility.

What tends to impose itself in relation to the modern ideal of autonomy are practices of heteronomy and passionate attraction. *Being young* becomes, as well, a new categorical imperative that entails ways of dressing, speaking, and taking care of one's body. Indeed, in his reflections Maffesoli alludes to a series of current juvenile phenomena that run from conceiving the enormous shopping centre as not only a functional place for simple purchase-sale transactions of products, but as a scenario for communion, through *raves* or *tecno-parties*, including the so-called *love parades*, to varied enthronings of fashion, astrology, soap operas ("eternities of pocket"), consuming *video-clips*, playing informatics games, the exacerbated utilization of cyberspace, the heyday of science fiction in movies or painting, the assuming of successive, ephemeral loves, a cult to the superfluous and frivolous, and *body art*, among so many other diffuse hedonisms.

Maffesoli posits a fundamental hypothesis: in the same way that modernity came to venerate the figure of the adult man, self-fulfilled, owner of himself and of nature, a man that exerts a principle of authority through prescriptive practices, what begins to dominate in nascent postmodernity is the myth of the *puer aeternus* – the eternal child – who in his permanent play imposes certain modes of being and of thinking. It is the presence of *Dionysius* that today extends itself over the grand cities of the West, revaluing the importance of the festive, of appearances, and of the notion of *destiny*. Existence, in effect, is seen as a succession of eternal instants. It is even possible to think that if work, in its productive, *crucifying* condition, was the sign of the modern period, the new cultural model will be that of play, of ludic activity with its dimensions of creativity. Thus, a tragic-ludic sentiment, a new, intense juvenile wisdom (as a kind of collective unconscious) seems to be returning with great strength to the daily life of the present, one that also always escapes from the logic of what *must be*. "The true life – Maffesoli affirms – exists everywhere except in the institutions (...) it has no projects because it has no precise objective. Hence the sharp aspect of its manifestations".[2]

Today brings a *re-enchantment of the world*, a new mythical time that can be appreciated, for example, in the current conjunction of the knight of lore and medieval legend with the image of the laser sword. If modernity privileged the future, then the contemporary period (like the decadence of Rome or the Renaissance) privileges the present. Modern western culture is oriented towards the future and the foundation of its action is in exteriority. All individual or social realization will thus be of the order of the *extensive,* inscribed in rationally-predictable *projects*, its vocation immanence. In a very distinct way, what seems to be accentuated today is the lived present suspended in the "fateful" dimension of existence that will be of the order of the *intense*, its vocation immanence.

In any case, the confrontation of destiny in the contemporary epoch does not mean, according to Maffesoli, simple resignation, but *a confrontation and a fury to live of undeniable social effects*: assuming destiny means the (tragic) acceptance of the paradoxical character of life, since it incites the dead to live, the "small deaths" of each day, and to "homoeopathically" integrate death into life as the best way to protect oneself and grow. What happens, then, is that life is lived "under the form of avidness" in an intense consummation that no longer seeks a presumed absolute, transcendental freedom but, rather, to exercise those small, relative, empirical *interstitial freedoms* on a daily basis. The tragic connotation lies in the acceptance of fatality as well as in the – often paroxysmal – incorporation of certain practices of pleasure.

Being becomes an *event* that sometimes arrives in a violent manner. Suddenly, for example, many young people display a kind of pagan exuberance that audaciously enjoys the vital present invaded by the freshness of the instant in all its intense transitoriness. Juvenile rebellions of multiform pleasure emerge that contravene the designs of any moralism of modernity, be it of an ideological, economic, or sexual order. A kind of *co-presence* in otherness is lived; a co-presence of variable modulations and intensity, but one that encompasses *being in its* everyday *becoming*, accentuating the potency of the impersonal, while what happens in many senses is that one is more actuated upon than actuating on one's own account. One often participates *magically* in the strange or new in an exercise that outstrips individual particularities. The existence and recognition of someone occur to the degree to which one's neighbour, or the social other, situationally endorses that existence and recognition. He who does not carry, in some way, the "scent of the clan" could be rejected or marginalized. But in any case, it is in this intensity and tragic-situational jubilation that the individual seems to fulfil her/himself in a *plus-being*.

Freedom and *necessity* are lived as a *contradictory* tension; that is, they are lived as a strange form of "conflictive harmony" that leads to the possibility of living a *plural I* (freeing oneself *from* oneself *in* the other) that affirms the sensitive existence of the here and now. This is an *ethics of the instant*: living in spite of it all. Thus, the new conception of social time is marked by the need to cope with destiny and *cyclical return*, the latter understood as the vital necessity of permanent regeneration. One desires an intense, sombre, vital, fascinating destiny, living an eternal present, a vitalism more-or-less conscious of itself, but one that ensures the persistence of being.

At all times, Maffesoli appeals to a *joy of the world* expressed in the power of *play* to configure present life as ephemeral, intense, ambivalent, with no pretension to dominate nature, history, society, or itself. A life that manifests an attitude more understanding than explicative, that implies greater relativism and a certain polytheism of values, and ponders an embodied, pluralist wisdom. In the face of the morosity of that which is instituted, what emerges is the rebellious joy of the institutor. "Rebellion against an abstract artificialism. Rebellion against a society of boredom. Rebellion against a programmed pseudo-life that leaves only a little space for adventure and the simple pleasure of existing. Rebellion, we must recall, alternative".[3] And rebellion, as well, of the imaginary. In this sense, Maffesoli recovers the importance of the world of appearances, of that *wisdom of seeming*, of that irruption of the image and exacerbation of the sensitice that can be appreciated in contemporary western societies. He also alludes to the notion of the *mask* to refer to the complexity of the roles and voices of real people immersed in diverse, changing situations.

Maffesoli speaks of a certain *viscosity* of the social through the emergence of co-identities; that is, networks and processes of hybridization in the world of today. He refers to a *social extasy* that, understood in the strict sense, implies exiting oneself to unite, paradoxically, with otherness and the world itself in all its heterogeneous character. The modern subject is today diluted in a constant *being-together*. The world is relativized, making it less dogmatic and more open. Being, therefore, cannot be understood as anything else than being with the other, or even being the other, in a return to a certain cosmogonic eroticism. Thus, Maffesoli underscores the notion of *passionate attraction* to emphasise the vitalist and creative attitude in today's world. In this epoch of the return of small gods, it becomes possible to assume a participation in the magical sense of things, people, and places, and to seek it out, touch it, and make multiform life with it. This participation is just as magical as it is contradictory; one rooted, *tragically*, in the present moment, in the bosom of the city (lived always as a succession of featured places). We are dealing with a *rejuvenation of the world*, a *re-imagining of it* by saying 'yes' (in spite of everything) to life. But then, what is to be thought of the moment of *dialogue*, of interlocution, in these circumstances? What changes and potentialities are involved?

In opposition to the dominant rationalism of modernity that impels individuals to transit through a shared project (political, economic, in-tellectual, or religious) that is adequate and *beneficial for all*, the postmodern life of the west seems to promote a *being together* that is much less am-bitious because it is immanent; a *being together* that – paradoxically – is prone to dispersion, one that comes branded by a kind of *sensitive* or *erotic reason* that vindicates a certain sentimental interest of the order of *empathy*, of desire, or of the imagination.[4] The *erotic reason* proposed by Maffesoli embodies the need for a principle that reconciles and contemplates, de-spite its constant contradictory becoming, the complex nature of reality in its active character.

Incapable of capturing the meticulous, imaginative, and symbolic as-pect of everyday experience, modern rationalism ignores the coincidence of opposites where completely antagonistic beings and phenomena can become intertwined and achieve a certain *existential conjugation*. By in-exorably seeking the essence and the constancy of the world, rationalism assumes, in contrast, the existence of indivisible, inalterable, linear, and univocal *units* for configuring and understanding collective life.

It is thus that *erotic knowledge* tends towards an acceptance of the world *as it is*, and not *as it should be*, it is a kind of interactive knowledge that incorporates within itself sombre moments and individual insufficiencies as well as the passions and lights that permit the development of some spaces of interpersonal relation or others. It is a thinking of *accompaniment*, a *metanoia* (that thinks on the side), opposed to a thinking of exclusion, a *paranoia* (that thinks in a dominant way). A *sensitive reason* acting in in-terlocution implies the incorporation of lived experience, of *common sense*, and of the affective, in the more-or-less unpredictable consecution of the encounter. It is not about the *dramatic* realization of a verbal exchange that derives from the *programme* stipulated by the order-words and prescrip-tions of modernity. It is not about the *efficient following* of principles, ideals, and methods that may have been outlined by discursive production and the intellectual and socio-emotional doings of institutions. By turning stagnant, these channellings of social praxis turn out to be arid and counterproductive for attesting to the intersubjective complexity and richness of shared verbal experience, especially in the presence of the emergent and unusual worlds of contemporary group life.

Sensitive reason demands a recognition of the very *desire* to know and relate oneself. He who desires something is he who does not possess that which he seeks; he who desires, desires what he does not have, something that does not coincide with himself. Here, the author alludes, once again, to otherness, to the strangeness of the other and of otherness, and to a subject that is not self-sufficient, one that in order to *be* requires the relation and encounter with those around him. Maffesoli opposes the figure of the expert thinker (possessor of knowledge) and proposes the figure of the contemplator desirous of mundane experience, in permanent tension with himself but, above all, not self-sufficient. In consequence, there will be a distancing with respect to the practice of a *dialogue* conceived as a methodical exercise of dialectic-scientific expansion, as an incisive interrogation, as an erudite response or affirmation, as an exclusion of *third parties* for the acquisition of *firm* knowledge.

What seems to be announced is a dialogue that seeks to separate itself from a *libido dominandi*; that is, from a knowledge linked to instrumental reasons and to the *universalizing* relations of power, in order to recover a *libido sciendi*, or "an erotic knowledge that loves the world it describes" because in this way "it purges itself of the general, of truth, of what is assumed to be just, the plausible and the possible of human situations can be glimpsed".[5] In reality, this is an *amorous*, relational, conjunctive *rationality* that is conscious of its own imperfection and unpredictability.

In such an experience of interlocution, metaphor will play a fundamental role because it must integrate – always provisionally – different meanings of the cognoscitive exercise associated with the encounter. Metaphor is located at the intersection of the *sensitive* milieu of social life and its codification in the act of knowing. It constitutes something like a *logos* revealed in images, a meaning converted into *form*. Here, I am thinking of a dialogue catalysed by a *stylistic* play of images that accentuates, *poetically*, the everyday and the symbolic, a more-or-less *useless* dialogue that involves a certain pre-eminence of the apparent and that assumes *form* (not only content) as a key dimension for its dispersed *realization*.

Maffesoli, in fact, distinguishes the notion of *form* from that of *formula*.[6] As a cultural vector, formula tends to look for *solutions*, it installs *certainties* by moving through a logic of the response. Form (and its philosophical expression denominated *formism*), in contrast, basks in the re-positing and multiplication of problems, while exploring, as well, the *conditions of possibility* that permit offering unfinished, specific, open responses situated in their concrete moment. Speaking in terms of *form* implies vindicating at each instant a certain *caricaturisation* of the real, a certain, more-or-less deliberate inappropriateness (unsuitability) regarding the tone of *objectivity* that the western discursive prescription demands for everyday exchanges. A shared speaking that questions in the act the tendency to relate in terms of *formula* and that, therefore, is not consequent with the constant mandate of *enlightened* clear expression. It is a shared speaking that comes to foment a certain variegation in what is said, one that can become affective, exaggerated, obscure, and *cavernous*, more than *diurnal* and efficacious.

Modernity, in both the foundations of political organization and the democratic ideal, as well as in the interpretative systems that it has developed, underscores the notion of *representation* for knowing the world in its *essential* and *universal* truths. Maffesoli suggests substituting *presentation* for representation, not as a simple linguistic change, but as a fundamental turn in the configuring of relations with the world itself and its knowledge. As epistemological and political attitude, *presentation allows it to be what it is* and becomes concerned with exalting the richness, dynamism, and vitality of the existential plexuses of the current moment. This does not impede – but actually favours – critical re-positionings with respect to that which is instituted and the tacit or explicit promotion of more-or-less interstitial or micro-political practices of rebellion and social or theoretical resistance. Presentation refuses to subscribe to the exercise of reducing, culling, or *perfecting* the heterogeneous reality in which we live. It is not possible to testify to the diversity of the world (nor transform it creatively) through the exclusive deployment of the rationalist gaze. It is not a question of thinking of univocal truths but, rather, of the paradoxes and interminable effervescences of social life.

As a result, a dialogue that occurs in these conditions emerges as an encounter of interlocution that does not tend towards *maturity* or plenitude in its adult, centred, or conclusive realization, but towards an unpredictable, corporeal, and imaginative *rejuvenation*. A dialogue that does not make an extreme hierarchization of the *content* to be developed but that delights in the *form* of its *unfinished realization*. It is also in this sense that I suggest the emergence of a *psychopoetics* in interlocution; that is, a dialogue that has less to do with an exercise in *education* than with an *initiatory* vocation; an interlocution that promotes zones of meaning not linked to any previously projected *objective* or *finality*, but that implies a moment of *rooting in the instant*, a world that is lived and that has been lived in the instant, zones of meaning that, moreover, are exhausted in the enunciative act itself to give rise to specific re-editions and variations.

A psychopoetic dialogue flees from the *dramatic*, linear time of the encounter, and from goals to be achieved, to constitute itself as a discontinuous exercise of the *presentation* of lived or imagined instants that are not entirely subject to the perspective of *control*, that do not seek to promote any specific effects *of development* in the play of interlocution itself. It is a dialogue that, in its constant reopening, does not pretend to (does not wish to and cannot always) explain what is said but, rather, *relive it*. This interlocution functions in that instant as a kind of *life-world* hinge. Due to its character, it opposes any *languid territory* and promotes a culture of invention that is somewhat *savage*. In another aspect, this event pre-supposes a certain *visceral* or incarnate inescapable wisdom, and with this, diverse affective participations and multiple, hybrid, *cosmic* identifications. It implies everyday verbal creations and variations, as well as a relative awareness of incompleteness and situational limits. But in any case, it inaugurates (though only fleetingly, imperfectly, and transitorily) a *being-together* for the discursive-interpersonal encounter itself.

The dialogical encounter is thus lived as a succession of passionate, thinking, creative, inter-corporeal, connected actualizations, whose *outcome* (if it exists) is unknown. This encounter does not always lead to the con-struction of the (grand) history of consensus or resolution; but interweaves small *errant* histories in their irreducible differences, with no obligatory precisions. From a *psychopoetic* perspective, "what communication is based upon is not so much a theoretical or informational content, as is the norm for the western tradition but, rather, a bond that is mysterious, tenuous and, for many, neither true nor false".[7] This tends to occur among groups of friends; its emergence is more likely, perhaps, in less institutionalized con-texts. This form of interlocution separates itself from universalisms, from functional certainties, and from the pretensions of definitiveness, to discover more-or-less enigmatic territories that gravitate in the encounter as an effect of the concomitant production of subjectivity.

This involves a mixture of ideas, objects, and people. It generates *fic-tions* of diverse kinds. It lives a clear *nomadism* in speech. It effectuates brusque turns of the rudder, and installs an unequal movement towards a certain perceptive and emotional *syncretism*. At that instant it returns to life, questioning in the act the immobility of *certainty*. It undoes one existential imprisonment or another. This shared, vitalist *psychopoetic* ex-pression can only occur when the speakers traverse the *present-existing-immanent world* – a crossing that can be difficult – perhaps vulnerable to nostalgia or to the moment of bitterness, but also, at any instant, jubilant.

In *psychopoetic* terms, dialoguing mean vindicating a *prosaic situationism*. It means *insolently* understanding the words of the interlocutor. This exercise cannot be the private ground of any *competent clergyman*; it is a form (ephemeral, intense) of speaking and of relating oneself that necessarily *escapes* from the designs of *intervention* ("professional", "authorized", or "resolutive") because it emerges *ordinarily*, since it is not planned, nor does it anticipate or intend any future benefits. But such encounters, in addition, emphasize in different ways the *re-creation* of the body: one gesticulates, dances, gets piercings or tattoos, dyes one's hair or procures a specific hairdo, introduces substances of diverse quality into the blood to experience their effects in groups, contacts others and interweaves one's own voice with the world through unpredictable corporeal (and technological) participations. One abandons messianic tones or hypocritical didacticisms except to sneer at them. One no longer dialogues for the *salvation* of anyone or to promote someone's health. One speaks not to judge but, in any case, to *link* what is said. Things are placed in relation, they are *relativised* and, at the same time, the alternative worlds of the interlocutor are made to appear as if on a stage.

It also happens that such experiences of verbal exchange turn out to be irreducible to any *conceptual* constriction. There is a separation of the abstract reasons that demand the *adequacy, rigour,* or *precision* associated with the need to *define* that which is expressed. In return, polysemy is accepted as an everyday practice of speech and appeals are often made to gratuitous exuberance. People dialogue in terms of a kind of *carnal reason* that promotes something like an *order* of the scattered, an order of the not delimited. In consequence, that dialogue (that in many ways renounces that which *must-be* said), lives an interesting *accidental* condition in the co-presence of the world and stimulates the emergence of the *de-ordered event* in its articulation with the inventive and complex becoming of social life.

Notes

1 See Maffesoli, M. (2001) *El instante eterno. El retorno de lo trágico en las sociedades posmodernas.* Buenos Aires: Paidós.
2 Maffesoli, M. *El instante eterno. El retorno de lo trágico en las sociedades posmodernas.* Ed. cit. p. 16.
3 Idem, p. 179.
4 See Maffesoli, M. (1996) *Elogio de la razón sensible. Una visión intuitiva del mundo contemporáneo.* Barcelona: Paidós, 1997.
5 Maffesoli, M. *Elogio de la razón sensible. Una visión intuitiva del mundo contemporáneo.* Ed. cit. pp. 16–17.
6 Idem, p. 114.
7 Maffesoli, M. *El instante eterno. El retorno de lo trágico en las sociedades posmodernas.* Ed. cit. p. 103.

6

POETICS OF DISORDER, ECCENTRICITY, AND TRANSIGNIFICATION

The notion of poiesis in ancient Greek philosophy

It is well-known that in ancient Greece the notion of *poiesis* – from the verb *poien* ("to make", "produce", or "fabricate") – was associated with the relative dimension of all creation; that is, to all *bringing into existence*. Hence, a *poiêma* is the "thing made" and the poet, *poiêtês*, is a "maker" linked through his activity to both the result sought and the creative process of its composition. Emilio Lledó holds that in Homer's literature the verb *poien* carries the sense of *making* something happen or *causing* it to happen,[1] but other meanings or connotations of the verb that have emerged (in the prosaist Herodotus, for example) associate it with *to celebrate* or *revel in* something, even *to consider something* or *take it something as*. Since Herodotus' time, it also appears in the sense of *to compose* and *to write*, linked to the poet's literary creation in accordance with the characteristics and properties attributed to that creation. In this sense, *poiesis* is conceived as *poetry*, a meaning that has endured through time.[2]

It turns out that *poiesis*, still in its initial meaning – as in reference to the "fabrication" or "production" of something concrete and material (wine, for example) – encounters an added meaning that has to do with *explaining* the process through which said production or elaboration takes place. For when speaking of *poiesis* it is important to think not only in terms of the component elements, but also of the *way* in which those elements have been composed, and the relation in which they participate. This relation alludes to the *logos* that has intervened in that reality to

DOI: 10.4324/9781003129295-6

conform it in the particular way in which it was, eventually, formed. The notion of *poiesis* cannot be reduced to the materiality of the object created for it entails, as well, considering the way in which its composition was achieved. *Poiesis* can thus be associated with the notion of *creation* as such, with action itself (as active process), but relatively autonomous with respect to the specific result of that action. Conceived in this way, *poiesis*

> is not be considered as the abstraction of a certain result, but as the process, the temporal development of an action that must culminate in an object (...). It does not, then, presuppose the existence of its object, nor can it be understood as the abstraction fixed in it; its abstraction is the 'not yet realisation' of the object towards which it tends, and its existence is as concrete as that of its result.[3]

In Heraclitus,[4] the verb *poien* is not concreted in an object but refers to the general *making* of human beings, to their *waking* works, everything that occurs during their waking-life, a *making* that is one ingredient of life in a state of wakefulness, a making that is a *making-with-the-logos*. The verb implies the sense of passing from not-being to being since that which is created *begins to exist* from the first instant of the creative action. *Poiesis* also takes on the sense of a "causal intervention of a qualitative modification"[5] or, perhaps better, the idea of *converting* something into something different. With respect to the relation between knowing and doing, *poiesis* presupposes a certain relation with practice and a certain *wisdom*.[6]

Democritus, meanwhile, suggests a conception of the poetic understood as *enthusiasm*. According to his view, poetic creation demands a certain, special state of intensity of anima: a certain *alteration* of animic stability; we might say a certain loss of *reason*. It sometimes occurs, Democritus affirms, that people's sensations and thoughts are produced by the influx into the body of *external images* or *éidola*. And it may happen that *éidola* enter people already *inflamed* by their own heat, by their agitated or nonsensical activity, and lead them to offer unusual reflections of greater signification, as occurs when *éidola* intervene in the nature of individuals with these tendencies, encountering there the most favourable or auspicious conditions for poetic creation. A poetic exercise thus requires not only the external influx of vivid images but also a certain special *internal* predisposition of the individual that fosters their appearance, a certain *sensitivity*. Poetic creation is not possible without *enthusiasm* seen as the instant at which the sensitized individual receives the influx of the divine *éidola* that allow him to contact or communicate with all that which differs from himself, thereby increasing his creativity.[7] The Sophists brought a rationalization of the notion of *poiesis*. Lledó affirms:

> If there is a common denominator that, imprecisely but constantly, underlies all opinions on poetry among the Greeks, from Homer to Plato, it is, without doubt, that this is a gift of a superior power that transcends the limits of the human being and through which [he] becomes totally absorbed. [But] the Sophists introduce a parenthesis in the conception of poetry. Plato would close this parenthesis and reunite once again with the ancient conceptions of 'divine possession' (…). This parenthesis of the Sophists provides a new element: reason.[8]

This means that the Sophists conceived poetic creation more the consequence of a rational construction – subject to rules like *rhythm* and *metrics* – than the product of a soul in trance like the individual enchanted by the divinities. This led Gorgias to define *poiesis* as word (*logos*) with metric (*metron*).[9] Poetic elevation is thus constituted by the formal-metric structure of a speech or discourse that differs from normal speech by displaying a certain mysterious tone that nears enchantment or *magic*. But it is not the supernatural that causes the poet's extasy; rather, it is *prestidigitation* as a constructive-rational exercise of verbal inventions thought beforehand and, hence, of a *technical* character. Here, *poiesis* is subsumed in the milieu of *logos*, converted into a *logos* with metrics, or perhaps in a part of the *logos* that produces certain effects since it can present the insignificant as something beautiful or provoke some emotion or another. As a result, poetic creation is inscribed as a *téchne*.

Plato, in turn, presented a kind of critique of Gorgias' thesis by questioning, in the dialogue *Ion*, whether poetic inspiration can really be associated with the terrain of *téchne*. There, Plato offers a reflection on poetry of a provisional character because it does not yet involves the key political connotation that this topic acquires in his *Republic*. The objective that Plato pursues here is just to demonstrate that in the trade of rhapsody, represented by Ion, no rigorous knowledge exists due, precisely, to the lack of *téchne*. The basis of this critique of poetry consists in denying that it implies knowledge concreted in (technically-established) procedures, rules, or norms that signal its practical, extended realization. Since it has no object of its own, nor any consistent realization, poetry cannot generate a poetic technique, which supposes a distancing from *true knowledge*, for this must be universal and applicable in all circumstances. Since there is no technique for its realization, the trade of poets – as rhapsodies

– becomes, at most, a *beautiful speaking* of one sole thing, but a speaking that is incapable of speaking well, or of explaining, not even minimally, all other things. Thus, the poet and his productions, indeed poetic inspiration itself, are not linked to technique, science, or wisdom but arise in the relatively irrational orbit of the *powers of deification*, of the divine strength that moves it. Finally, the poet who produces *beautiful songs* is not "in his reason", but dominated by all that is harmonious and rhythmic. He loses his serenity and intelligence and can no longer see reality itself, know it, or express it. He becomes passionate, living deceived by the madness of the Muses.[10] At another moment, however, somewhat in contradiction to the foregoing, Plato described the poet – in the mouth of Socrates – as someone extremely sensitive, and poetry (delirium inspired by the gods) as something that allows access to knowledge and the understanding of the future.[11] Nonetheless, according to Lledó's explanation, Plato apparently wished to "take gravity and power away from the poetic opus, reduce it to a delicate game, an irrational moment of the spirit, estranged as such from all knowledge and, in consequence, incapable of teaching anything or of exercising any educational function".[12]

In his *Republic*, Plato elaborated a direct reprobation of poetry in which he conceives of the poet as lacking *intelligence* and the capacity to communicate true knowledge. Because he enters a state of *poetic trance* he cannot be a teacher or educator of the people. Here, the poet is closer to *seer*, even *prophet*, than *philosopher*. His territory is particularity and the contingent, sensitive, and emotional life, but not that of *thought* which produces *universal* knowledge through access to *ideas*. "Poetry is the faithful painting of animated nature, and not the reasoned analysis of a supraphysical existence, created through rarification of reality. In this sense poetry points towards the multiple".[13] When the poet creates his works *alienated* by the divinity, inspired by Muses, he is, in one way or another, *outside of himself*; his creation is *impulsive* in nature, not the result of a *technique*. For this reason, the poet cannot *explain* his compositions. This is what Plato critiques: a product that has not been created through a conscious construction of a technical order that presupposes a prior rationality.

But this brings us to the question of whether it is more convenient to accept or reject the poetry of the new *Polis*,[14] but also opens a critique of poetry itself from the perspective of the theory of ideas. Poetic work is assumed, in effect, in its *corrupting* function of thought. For Plato, poets speak from a plane that is not in contact with things in themselves. They do not *know* what they say, but are only *imitators* of the world. Since they do not address *truth*, they must be combatted. They are not *authentic* creators, not like the artisans that fabricate objects in conformity with an idea, because they are artifices of *all manner of objects, even of themselves,* though only in terms of *appearance.*[15] They offer *images* of reality, but not its *essences.* Poets speak of thinks distant from true reality because they are only concerned with reproducing or (perhaps) *recreating* elements that pertain to the milieu of the perceptible, but do not approach the domain of *ideas.* They interpret human values but without so much as brushing up against *truth.*[16] The word of the poet does not reveal *being,* does not allude to the ontological content of the world, but only exposes appearances in their *chromatism.* The word of the poet is not oriented towards the *understanding* of things, but to celebrating the *appearance* of things in their intense colouring, in a rhythmic, harmonious way with not a care for the truth it expresses, only for the enchantment, fascination, and beauty it produces.[17] In this regard, Lledó comments:

> Poetic language thus encloses, in itself, that magic power capable of separating he who listens to it from all rational consideration; and it exercises this not for an artificiality, but due to its very nature (...). The word poetic holds within itself, and as such, this strength that goes beyond the purely significative field (*logos*) and gives it a new and diverse perspective.[18]

Plato distinguishes two parts of the soul: one rational, the other irrational. Poetry affects the soul and can modify it, change moods, generate diverse emotions, but these modifications occur precisely in relation to the *irrational* part of the soul, that deceptive, illusory domain marked by *equivocation,* incapable of accurately perceiving reality for it does not discern the true *being* of things because it escapes reason and lives without control. As a result, those who deliver their soul to poetic emotion contravene the ideal of the citizen of the new *Polis,* one who must govern himself by reason and by law,[19] without the contradictions and raptures of passion. The poet is a *political* collaborator of the irrational part of the soul who speaks to that irrational part through his creations. Therefore, he *must* not be admitted into the city[20] unless he renounces any possible educational function and devotes himself solely to singing hymns to the gods.

The poetic is associated not with serene wisdom, nor with the intellectual, objective, serious assumption of reality, but to the inventive, enthusiastic interpretation of the world. It tends more towards the mythical than the logical. The poetic has to do with a certain *madness,* a certain *delirium* that does not describe, narrate, or make *history,* but only *recreates, extols, intensifies, colours* events. It configures new worlds by disfiguring the world itself. It does not probe deeply, but makes its subject material more *complex* and *unpredictable*. It is not directed towards knowledge but to a dynamized, changing realization of the world. The poetic does not separate itself intellectually from the world, but imbricates with it. It does not pretend to respect the conditions and characteristics of the *object* so as to study it, but transforms or modifies it as part of its more-or-less *irreverent* creative impulse. The poetic alludes not to the objective formalization of relations with the world, but to a chromatic, hetero-geneous reinvention of those relations. The appearance and movement of the *poetic object* is not possible, then, without the poetic impulse itself; that is, without the protection of *poiesis*.

In political terms, Plato's impugnation of poets is linked to the cri-terion that an unbridled freedom that succeeds in escaping from any *authority* constitutes something worse than *any government*.[21] The poet disdains authority and order, lets himself be carried away by sensory pleasures, *subverts* the norms and precepts of what is reasonable and so perniciously influences the multitude. It is, therefore, necessary to banish poets, not solely on metaphysical or ontological grounds (alluding to poetry's inability to accede to the true *being* of things) but, above all, *on political grounds* (alluding to the impugnation of *unbridled* practices of freedom). What Plato cannot pardon is the possible rupture of a principle of a supreme order: the *authority* of the State. Legislation must impede poets from *composing* whatever may occur to them to ensure that no expressions contrary to the laws appear, expressions that by their very nature damage the city.[22]

This counterposition between *poiesis* and law (or *poet* and *legislator*) occurs precisely because *poiesis* implies *creation* while law implies *con-servation*. If the poetic involves production, understood as the passage of an entity from *not being* to *being*, then law, in contrast, constitutes the confirmation of those realities, the subjection of entities to a certain *or-dering* and the regulation of their consequent behaviours. Law tends to delimit realities, while *poiesis* lives by transgressing boundaries. Poetic creation is not subject to norms and, therefore, ceases to be a logical or *reasonable* practice. Those who legislate cannot say two different or op-posed things with respect to the same object, they are obliged *to define*. The poet, in contrast, does not legislate, but *opens* different worlds, names things in a distinct way, does not *define* the object but *reinvents* it, *diversifies* it. Plato condemns the *free* labour of the poet and his (irreverently) creative activity, while firmly maintaining that all creation must be subject to the state and its legislation.[23]

Eccentricity and the deforming adventure of the senses

I subscribe to the idea that when speaking, the exercise of continuous expression tends to separate constantly from its (supposed) *command centre*; that is to say that dialogue can unfold as an active process of *decentring* (escape) from any prescriptive nucleus of the initial signification of the encounter. To the extent that this occurs, dialogue becomes *eccentric* by deviating and multiplying in new aspects thereby betraying, disattending, or breaching in a certain way its structuring duty. In the process of acceding to eccentricity, dialogue passes through a *conversational* moment, but its movement does not necessarily conclude in that instant; rather, through a kind of creative disintegration of speech, *something comes to happen*. A *mixture of bodies* is produced and with it some kind of *incorporeal transformations* or another that, as we know, Deleuze and Guattari associate with the *act of language*, with the *transformation of realities*. The dialogue that is de-centred (that becomes eccentric) constitutes a *prism* that cracks to bring about the event (as happens, perhaps, with the *decomposition of light*). Eccentricity in dialogue produces new realities.

Dialogue-conversation comes about as part of what could be denominated an *immanent journey*. The subject in interlocution must be transformed into *homo viator*. "We are *on the way* – Joan-Carles Mèlich writes – in constant change, in incessant transformation, though not in absolute transformation, for (...) *there is nothing absolute in human life*".[24] In effect, through everyday dialogue (in all its complexity, interconnections, and variations), the subject is able to see, hear, and enunciate worlds immersed in something like an interminable journey towards a given territory of *order* or (changing) configuration of things. The subject (always in a network) sees, hears, and enunciates worlds in a journey full of unpredictable turns and transformations. Where is the subject who sees, hears, and enunciates such *worlds* going?; or, perhaps better, what is the destination of those *worlds* that transit through the intimacy of the subject who sees, hears, and enunciates them? José Lezama Lima seems to respond: "(...) a landscape goes towards a meaning, an interpretation, or a simple hermeneutics, to later go towards its reconstruction, which is definitively what marks its efficacy or disuse, its orderly force or its muted echo, which is its historical vision".[25] Whatever it may be that a subject sees, hears, learns, and speaks, he does so during an inexorable journey because human life is nothing more than a continuous transiting, a moving through the cultural and corporal geography of existence.

The subject becomes related to, and imbricated with, the world in becoming when he unstoppably abandons some primary home. In my view, relating to the changing world entails that journey through which one leaves, forever and at each instant, some anterior condition. This is a journey that at every moment produces *the loss of a certain condition/stay/ form/state*, only to create another, new, *condition/stay/form/state* whose birth is precisely the turn of its disappearance. Each world thus emerges in the act of dying. Expressed in another manner, each world is wrecked in the very act of being born, in its ill-timed irruption before the subject's eyes, ears, and word. Each existential plexus results from a *hallucinatory*, often terrible, *ride*.

The subject comes to relate to, and mix with, his surroundings as he produces new visibilities and discourses to contribute to the metamorphosis of that environment. He acts as a *metaphorical and imaginative subject* who produces new experiences and new worlds out of what he is given. He reads, writes, speaks, and feels worlds through metaphors and images constituted by configurations more-or-less integrated into the context. This is why the event that the subject lives can never be conceived as "pure fact", nor can the object be conceived in its supposed "purity", because any possible event or object immediately involves immense resonances of diverse meaning. The subject converts the event in metaphor, in a new vision, new voices, new life; in unison, those metaphors, visions, voices, and lives disappear in the heat of the events, opening the way to others, and this goes on successively.

The subject in interlocution becomes a prism that transforms and combines nature and culture; perception and imagination (all through its *errant* condition as well):

> If I say stone, we are in the dominions of a natural entity, but if I say the stone where Mario cried in the ruins of Carthage, we are constituting a cultural entity of solid gravitation. Warp strength and gravitation characterise that space counterpointed by the imago, which provides the extension to where that space has animist strength in relation to those entities.[26]

The subject occupies the space of the world in order to organize it; to imagine it in distinct configurations of *saying*; to create it in the heat of the *animist counterpoint* that emerges with respect to the events he lives. "With time (...) it will become manifestly impossible to employ any technique that is not that of 'fiction'".[27] All discursive expression, any narration or description of the world, dialogued or not, constitutes in this sense the specific movement of a *fiction*. This is how each subject *realises* his journey through life, where it soon expresses "the relief of its acquisitions".[28] All realism creates its own reality. Each subject lives submerged in the discursive ocean of culture.

The event, in turn, also occupies the space *of the* subject in order to organize it, to invent it in a different way. The event forms an *image* for the subject, creates the subject, *speaks* it in a particular way. Thus, the subject is also *spoken*, invented, created by the event. The subject both speaks and is spoken, creates and is created, lives in an ongoing reconstruction of its existential plexuses, actively produces its expression amidst a framework with the world. I can express this as follows: the speaker produces its subjective expression in a constant reinventing of the world; and at the same time the world produces its objective expression in a constant reinventing of the speaker.

The *truth* of an event, its very existence, bonds to the production of culturally- and discursively-determined meanings. The event emerges into the interior of a material-discursive sphere (a natural-social-imaginary world) in which the subject *travels*, where it achieves its *reality*, and where one notices that its progress is halted. An event without this sphere that confirms it (deciphers it), becomes *undecipherable*. Lezama writes:

> When in '*La chanson de Roland*' it is stated with great precision that [during] the conquest of Zaragoza Charlemagne was two hundred and twenty years old; when we see that the Saracens pledged [loyalty] to Apollo and Mohammad; when it is said that Roldán, upon defeating an Arab, 'pulled out his soul with the point of his spear', these are all events gravitated by the era of Charlemagne, by a kind of hypostasized imagination.[29]

Truth, then, will be *imaginative* while the subject shoots, from his socio-discursive platform, the powerful arrow that *unveils* a world; that forces it to emerge from its hiding place and come into presence; that obliges it to pass from *not being* to the *being* of a certain form and at a certain instant an "arrow in flight that we cannot return to the bow".[30] The arrow of which I speak is the *poetic* one. But the created world returns upon the subject itself with its own strength; infiltrates its images (like Democritus' *éidola*) into the body and voice of the speaker; forms it, situates it and, in a certain way, *controls* it. Hence, subject and world do not maintain a link of subordination (antecedent-derived) in one direction or the other, but constitute, in effect, two differentiated moments of socio-natural becoming through whose trance collective existence produces its reliefs and acquires dissimilar meanings. Each speaker is the unrepeatable expression of the material-imaginative framework that is woven with the world. Each speaker produces permanent mutations and alterations with respect to the real and with respect to his own life trajectory, such that what results is, precisely, that each speaker in his interaction *is, definitively, never the same.*

In this domain what may sometimes occur is a dialogue prone to deviations, to involving an appetite for inventions. A dialogue that *incorporates* the landscapes of audacity and mobilizes the generating potency of some other *imaginative condition/stay/form/state.* A dialogue that ceases to be a centred exercise in order to dedicate itself to cutting, zigzaggedly and erratically, intersubjective distances. This is a *dialogue-pirate* that carries adventure in its blood, that drinks from amazement, that seeks *something* it has never known. Or, perhaps better, a *dialogue-fiesta* ruled by the intoxicating desire of interwoven music and banquet. "We eat – Serres now writes – drink to the health of some and others, share tobacco, ending when an invisible hand writes on the wall the unknown words of death".[31]

A *psychopoetic* dialogue is one that, even in its disorder (or perhaps thanks to it) promotes a *transporting of oneself to another life,*[32] a loose, open, free dialogue that has no fear of, nor rejects, variegation. A dialogue that detaches from itself (as a more-or-less prescribed script) in an effort to foster the shifting of the world to another place, a place unplanned; in other words, a dialogue that travels with the interlocutors in the act of abandoning earlier *condition/stay/form/state* to accede to others; of opening new affective dimensions of word and action in detriment to previous identitary fixations. In psychopoetics, Juan is *Juan-at-the-same-time-as-he-ceases-to-be-him*: Juan abandons himself, travels to transform himself in other thing(s) through the *idiographic* effervescence of the encounter itself. In this way, the personal subject bears the unpredictable sign of *being lost* in its heterogeneous interconnection (Sloterdijk has said that humans are beings who are "a little lost").[33] He travels and connects in order to *cease to be himself.* Withdrawing from that journey –remaining petrified at some point – means certain symbolic *death* that, however, can also be extended, unequally, in the domain of interaction. The personal subject is reborn intermingled with the world, and *lives dying* in that (immanent) journey of *de-subjection.*

According to Claudio Magris,[34] there are two ways to conceive a *journey*: on the one hand, the *journey of formation* in which the protagonist returns home, returns to the setting-off point in conditions of greater maturity enriched in some way by life (the case of Ulysses in the *Odyssey* is paradigmatic); on the other, is the *journey of deformation*, whose fundamental characteristic is that the protagonist never returns home, but gets lost along the way (an example could be the figure of "Ulrich", the principle antihero of Robert Musil's *The Man without Qualities*).[35] In this regard, I consider that the exercise of dialogue fomented under the aegis of the practice of psychological or pedagogical intervention characteristic of the normalizing apparatuses of modernity generally promotes (or in many cases at least aspires to achieve) *journeys of formation*. This is a dialogue directed towards the specific conformation of the subject in accordance with the requirements of the political administration of capitalism: a practice of interlocution oriented technically towards returning the subject to itself, devoted to consolidating the functional individual and/or to its full *realisation* in a certain configuration of knowledges and forms of being, feeling, and acting. What psychopoetics foments, in contrast, are *journeys of deformation*: dialogues that subvert the vectors of normalization and the functional development of institutions to open, in constant creative escape and dispersion (and in the tacit or explicit negation of educational, therapeutic, or analytical objectives) other possibilities of relation, other existential plexuses, as interstitial as they are unusual, as chromatic as they are useless, and that, moreover, renounce beforehand the formative mandate of that return (*i.e.*, of that consolidation) of those involved with respect to themselves in a key of maturity, social competitivity, or personal plenitude.

Psychopoetics impugns all substantial, solidified, or *idealised* formulations of the world or of itself, associated with some apparatuses of prescription or of order-word or others (this in no way invalidates the adoption of political positions by interlocutors in accordance with experience and situation). In this regard, the key aspect is that the interlocutors do not have to be, nor have to realize, any preconceived *essence*, do not have to fulfil more-or-less transcendent objectives, do not have to advance through any presumed collective or individual historical vocation, do not necessarily have to follow any *programmed destiny*. Its distinguishing mark is provisionality, the possibility to always respond in a different way. This is the critical vindication of plurality and of the unfinished in contrast to the *reglementary* practice of definitive, complete expression. If a supposed *ideal* dialogue sets out (as Serres explains)[36] to *eliminate background noise*; if in Platonic terms said dialogue is directed towards *episteme* and not *doxa*; if that exercise, in the spirit of Buber, presupposes an ethical-moral vocation through the *recognition of the other as person*[37]; then, in contrast, a psychopoetic dialogue must be described as a more-or-less *disobedient*, more-or-less *irresponsible*, exercise that does not know or recognize as much as it *invents*; that does not eliminate, but mixes in with the background noise; that delights in the festive differing of opinions.

The psychopoetic encounter should produce a decentring of identity, a propensity towards the *deforming* turn of the participants with respect to their surroundings and themselves. In its becoming, psychopoetics implies an exercise of interlocution that produces *unanticipated* results for the realization of the encounter. It involves a permanent potential for surprise in the event of sense. It implies various *apertures* to unexpected frameworks. It proposes interpretations that permit "remaining open to an always uncertain possibility [one] never completely controllable or plannable".[38] It thus flees from authorised or foreseen certainties. It avoids determinist definitions unless to dethrone and reject them in a critical or parodic key. A psychopoetic dialogue differs from the dialogue produced in psychological intervention because the latter (as institutionalized praxis) tends, sooner or later in my view, towards deterministic formulation, definitory closure, the prescriptive word, the resolution of varied conflicts or situations, and the more-or-less efficient performance of directed actions.

The practices of dialogical interlocution produced in the interventive activity of institutions, in contrast to the fine crafting of intersubjective differences, tend towards what, to paraphrase Joan-Carles Mèlich, I can denominate a *techno-psychological monomythism*[39]; that is, a more-or-less programmed tendency to enthrone the criteria of thought and action that circulate in institutionalized dialogue, seeking to ensure that the prescriptive – we might say, *formative* – vectors of subjection in modernity are followed. Practices intended to deny or minimize the domain of the contingent, while absolutising, or maximizing, in distinct ways, the domain of the presumed *capacity of choice* and *independence* of the subject in accordance with the dominant universe of knowledge and power.[40] Perhaps one of the most formidable manifestations in this sense appears with the advance of all those well-dressed (nefarious) preachers of *excellence* and *self-improvement* whose proposals emphasize, for example, that escaping from poverty is a simple question of individual *choice*.

Techno-psychological monomythism tends towards *indoctrination*, not freedom, for every time that a pedagogue, psychologist, psychoanalyst, or psychotherapist suspends or erases from his dialogue with the subject the critical attitude with respect to that which is established, or impedes any *political conscientisation* of the contingent, provisional, unfinished, fragile, bitter, laughter, the finite, or the unpredictable, that *intervener* is acting in the service of hegemony and of a subtle kind of totalitarianism. In effect, psychological intervention operates through the re-productive adaptation of the subject to the environment, and tends to link *identity* to a certain consistency in the realization of some social *functions* or others. The aim is not only to promote a *functional* subject, but to convert that subject into a *functionary* of the system, bereft of broad margins for improvisation, op-positional creativity, or irreverent initiative. The idea is to ensure (at all costs) the endurance of a world without ruptures, fissures, disobedience, subversions. Dis-harmony is not tolerated, the subject must be happily subjected to an obligatory *harmonisation* with the positive functioning of the social machinery.

Thus it is that, immersed in the territory of specialization, of optimal performance, and of efficiency as order-word, the exercise of dialogue does not favour the assumption of multiplicity, but fosters a flattening of subjective reliefs, eludes the experience of metamorphosis, seeking always to advance smoothly –infallibly – as if on railroad tracks. Psychopoetics constitutes, precisely, the political, interstitial, minoritarian negation (by rebelling – and revealing itself – before such enunciative prescriptions) of all those structuring aspects of the technical dialogue that characterises institutional reproducibility. Psychopoetics implies a critical fiesta of senses, not the uniformity of objectives, sustained not by *programming* but by *desire*. That is why this *deforming dialogue* does not fit (though it may appear as a stowaway on the ship of normalized interlocution) into the diverse socio-discursive apparatuses entrusted with reproducing and transmitting senses, including the various types of psychotherapies, psy-chological, sexual, vocational, or educational orientation, teaching practices of diverse kinds, or self-improvement and "self-help" groups. Psychopoetics becomes *impertinent*, subverting in the act that conservative-technical-economic-moralistic-prescriptive-conceptual character that, as a fundamental sign, attends and supports the link with others in the institutionalized dialogue (speaking with "effectivity" and speaking "correctly" because "nothing is gratuitous in the *competitive* world in which one lives") with the function of reducing the complexity of the contingent and, above all, attempting *to control events*.

In its *verbal adventure*, psychopoetics often mocks the hieratic discourse of definitiveness. Psychopoetics tends to impede a centred, objective perception of the environment, tends to distrust any essentialist or *re-petitive* vocation, appealing, rather, to the experiential and inventive do-main of speech. It involves the ongoing transformation of the speakers' thinking and emotionality. *Psychopoetic reason* is *impure, fragmentary, mul-tiple, fetishist*. It does not aspire to validation, does not claim verifiability of what is said, its importance perhaps *testimonial, uncertain*. Its realization is, thus, imperfect, and vulnerable. Participants live a kind of discursive-corporal collusion which fosters that things *occur* in their diversity of senses. For this reason, these deforming dialogues of psychopoetics tend towards more-or-less radical innovations in enunciation, involve critiques of established values, and vindicate an incessant changing of the *real* world through imagination. Disruptive, intense, more-or-less uncontrollable, strange at times, laughable, disconcerting, polyphonic, desirous, anti-programmatic; psychopoetics emerges now and then in interlocution, and goes out of its way to find *difference*; though inevitably, together with the re-enchantments it produces, it often proceeds joined, as well, to *disenchantment*. But in any case, psychopoetics seems to revive *a form of interlocution in which power is decomposed in terms of possibility.*

Transignification and the inventive turn

While the notion of language is generally related semiotically to the instituted *order of reality*, its permanent dynamism and renovation, and its diverse possibilities of meaning and sense in its specific uses and rules, we must point out that language always manifests itself in *concrete languages*; that is, specific linguistic formations differentiated by the characteristics of their associated activities and the socio-material ways of life of each case. These are open, changing sub-systems of acts and expressions of speech itself in all its possibilities of situational concretion within the context of its plurality. What occurs is that the verbal matter of concrete languages is not reduced to constituting a *tool* for the consecution of the goals of some interventive activities (though we must admit that those verbal processes imply a certain relative *availability* or *determinability* for the consecution of diverse goals that are the product of their historical sedimentation and the social relations that accompany the concrete uses and play of language itself).[41] In any case, concrete languages and their everyday exchange constitute the base upon which all verbal *re-composition*, all discursive creation, and all new production of subjectivity, is generated in the domain of social bonds.

Psychopoetics emerges, above all, because it constitutes one of the possibilities of concrete languages in everyday relations or exchange. Exchanges that, moreover, function *online* with the social materiality of the world. Psychopoetics constitutes a generation of signification and meanings and a configuration of existential plexuses in the interlocution associated with unrepeatable affective connections of the encounter. The emergence of psychopoetics depends, on the one hand, on the verbal matter current in the concrete languages involved in the dialogue, with their specific relations and connotations but, on the other, also on the *vital event* that may take place in said encounter: the event of the creative recomposition of the *very states of things* (or states of reality) that are acting in that instant. Psychopoetics implies an imaginative-verbal combination of confronted or exchanged expressions by virtue of which the permanence of instituted speech is impugned and situations are opened that, in some way, subvert the ordinary or normal meanings of those expressions (contrarily, a dialogue that clings to its semantic load, that tends to close itself in a conformation of meanings, does not favour the emergence of psychopoetics). For these reasons, in psychopoetics any significant component is necessarily provisional or transitory. Its illative condition is unstable. It goes beyond the domain of *signification* to move towards *meaning*, always renewed.

Psychopoetics does not burst forth as a natural derivation of the dialogical encounter; rather, it entails a rupture with ideal semantic dialogue, implies an event that goes beyond the merely functional scope of the interlocution. The psychopoetic event tends to escape from linguistic prescription, is not reduced to a play *of the* language, but involves instead – as Josu Landa affirms with respect to the poetic event – a "peculiar becoming of a certain kind of play *in* languages".[42] Psychopoetics does, indeed, constitute a form of interlocution that on the basis of, and despite, its significative functions (semantic load) subverts those functions when it encounters favourable conditions to do so. It is an interlocution that inaugurates realities distinct from the *order of the signification*: one separated by moments from the logical-discursive prescription of speech, thus renouncing compliance with *certainties* and the ideal transmission of illative contents as *messages*. In other words, psychopoetics does not appeal, fully, to the truth of what is said. This is precisely the opposite focus to the perspective of interventive dialogue, which converts interlocution into a means (of a technical-scientific-professional order) for installing in participants theoretical *truths* and promoting more-or-less sophisticated practices of normalization, assistance, and/or *development*.

Psychopoetic dialogue has a connection of a *tentative* character with the rationality that operates in established languages. Its emergence supposes the more-or-less arbitrary utilization of terms and expressions that, placed together, stray from their literal meanings to accentuate unusual connotations according to the special, unrepeatable situation of the interlocution itself. To the extent that the expressions of the dialogue remit to signification as such – that is, adhere to their condition of *normal* discourse, as occurs predominantly in discursive activity – the possibility of *psychopoetic realities* is excluded. Psychopoetics eludes univocity and the literal condition of that which is spoken. It does not endorse precise or substantial correspondences between the word that is spoken and that which is named. It creates alternate worlds in an oscillating zone of linking-unlinking with respect to the semantic-pragmatic condition of verbal exchange; a zone of interlocution in which, of course, the discursive uses current in that concrete historical moment continue to participate decisively. While the dialogue of intervention strives to consolidate its nexuses with meaning, psychopoetics tends to undo those nexuses. For this reason, psychopoetics in its functional discontinuity with respect to discursive conventions becomes more-or-less creative and unpredictable.

What psychopoetics transforms, therefore, is the *normalised* manner in which concrete languages are presented in dialogue. It potentiates new alternatives of movement for those languages through unexpected variants of the vertebration of expressions in an ongoing correlation with the socially-determined interactive life of the interlocutors ("dialoguers") themselves. We might say that psychopoetics emerges from the *alterations* of the social relation occasioned by the novel or inventive verbal articulation in the domain of the dialogical encounter. There is, in psychopoetics, a tendency to dismiss all linguistic essentialism (since it does not necessarily identify any contained significance with one predetermined function or another). New possibilities for the *realisation* of dialogical interaction arise in accordance with the specific situation. The orders of reality instituted by dominant discourses are often relatively disobeyed, and interlocution is assumed as an experience freed from the imperative (tacit or explicit) of *conclusion*. Psychopoetics *denaturalises* the verbal matter of the interlocution and differentiates itself from a normalized dialogue because it provides a productive alteration of expressions. This is an imaginative, emotional differentiation compared to the *indifference* of the discursive development.

A key condition for the emergence of psychopoetic dialogue consists in the process thanks to which what occurs first is a *designification* of the verbal matter (a speech that *denies* the semantic components of what is said) in order to open, afterwards, a domain of reality distinct from the order of the discourse. In Landa's reflection:

> It is impossible to know of what the word is capable, but [we can] reasonably sustain the idea that it must desist from its normal nexuses with the world so that it can make way for another class of connections, like those implied in the word in the poetic situation.

> There is – expressed in Hegelian style – a kind of cunning in the word by virtue of which it can be articulated according to formations and be given in conformity with situations that allow it to free itself from its usual determinations.[43]

This designification implies an exit from the commonly accepted literality in interlocution; that is, a relative rupturing of that which is expressed from its habitual references in reality; but simultaneously, a moment of the *transignification* of that which is said towards the immanent possibility of the *event* must also occur. Interlocution becomes psychopoetics to the degree that it produces a situational and inventive fissure in the continuity of the restraints characteristic of the illation of dialogue itself; or, perhaps better, to the extent that an *extra-limitation* of that which the expression utilized *normally* implies occurs.

Transignification cannot be reduced to the mere re-assignation of meanings to certain words or expressions. Rather, it implies crossing the limits of operative discourses to remake (or recompose) the social relations that exist with whomever the interaction takes place. Recomposing relations in the sense of creating novel existential plexuses; that is, provoking *poetic* effects in the field of intersubjectivity. Psychopoetics then, as a space of transignification, supposes a complex re-editing of interpersonal relations in the dialogical-conversational encounter. A vertebration of inventive actions in speech. A transit from more-or-less *static* expressive uses (those that deploy stable, reiterated meanings and senses and constitute a kind of *platform of meaning*) towards other *dynamics* or extraordinary ones (that incorporate translational, substitutive, and/or revocatory movements of existing semantic-pragmatic orders). Even so, all creativity linked to an *extraordinary* discursive production in dialogue will necessarily be marked by current expressive uses – instituted socially and communitarially – that in their function as a significative platform or base intervene in the delimitation, specific articulation, scope, and particular modes in which the inventive *cunning* of speech occurs in that dialogical encounter.

Psychopoetics requires a certain expressive *audacity* on the part of its participants, an irreverent handling of the meanings and a production of peregrine, surprising, strange, or amusing senses that goes beyond everyday stipulations. "Concretely – Landa writes – languages house the possibility of verbal compositions that stand above the regularities of the dynamics [of language]. This entails a negation of the conventions of meaning and sense as the fundamental condition (...)". However, this same author specifies that

The other necessary condition is pertinence to the semantic exchanges to which that negation opens the way. To allude to a rather vulgar example, there could not be much pertinence in the attempt to make the term 'bacon' into a metaphor of the word 'velocity'. The extraordinary metaphoric (that is, the suspension of linguistic normalcy by metaphor) must be accompanied by a certain *adaequatio* among the interchangeable meanings.[44]

The psychopoetic rupture in interlocution can never, therefore, be *total*; it entails expressions that shed themselves of their usual meanings, that open distinct terrains in the production of senses, that *de-signify* the verbal matter and accede to a *transignificant* dimension, but that cannot absolutise their *renunciation* or *disobedience* to those illative prescriptions (of minimal referential coherence) present in ordinary verbal exchanges.

In addition to the foregoing, the psychopoetic condition in speech cannot be understood as a *means* for the intentional achievement of other, subsequent goals. It does not constitute a predictable resource for acceding to a knowledge, nor for explaining something, transmitting values, promoting respect for, and recognition of, the other interlocutor, or any other operation of the kind; that is, operations of an *interventive* nature. This transpires because the psychopoetic condition involves a certain *transgression* of the semantic and pragmatic unfolding of languages and because it alters or distances itself from verbal functions of discursive normalization and automatism in speech. Psychopoetics may, perhaps, be initiated by some expressive *gimmick* that opens, at a given instant, the possibility of new modes of relating to concrete languages: estrangement of the topics addressed; placing *things* and *words* in unhabitual networks; infractions of the practical codes of speech; frustrating modes of recurrent speech; abandoning predictable regularities in interlocution. Psychopoetics asserts its inventions and introduces distinct interstitial and transitory worlds into the encounter, thus exciting disquietude, and sedition against all operative prescription of the filtered *intervention* in dialogue, and suddenly raising up the passions of participants.

Psychopoetics emerges on the interminable discoursing of the word but requires, in turn, a situational base and a milieu of intersubjective relations that favour it. It is never a *creatio ex nihilo*. It constitutes a productive tension or tightness between extended *verbality* and the subversion of such *normalising* determinations upon interacting. But whatever the case, its emergence will be linked to its *own context of realisation* that includes, in my view, some objects and material resources articulated with the doings of the interlocuters (dialoguers), or others, certain micro-cultural relations of socialization and, of course, a certain complex connection of corporealities and subjectivities that concur (at least momentarily) with the verbal-inventive encounter in question. Psychopoetic dialogue thus involves an always unfinished, concrete *space-situation* of realization, a space made up of a network of heterogeneous links between people and things (micro-communities) more-or-less well-disposed towards exchanging proposals and expressions and to verbal-creative action in accordance with the circumstances and conditions of the encounter.

In its activation, psychopoetics involves all participations (though differentiated) of those who sustain this form of interlocution. There is no room for passive subjects in this process. The things said in this type of encounter will be, for better or worse, everyone's *affair*. But everything spoken in such a conversational space implies expressions transited by a creative activity linked to, and sustained by, a kind of *energetic* realization of the word. Each subject contributes some enunciative productions – or others – not uniformized in their presentation but that, even in their specific interweaving with the contributions of the other people, maintain a certain autonomy of style, a certain character of unrepeatable *authorship*. Even so, no psychopoetic production in interlocution is, or can ever be, *absolute* in its *originality*, because it is never exempt from diverse socio-discursive determinations characteristic of the historical-concrete situation and, moreover, because it always requires a socio-material field, milieu, or network of relations that confer sense beyond the aforementioned originality or character of authorship.

In any case, there will be no unitary or *unconditioned* mode of living the psychopoetic experience in interlocution. Although that encounter produces unrepeatable intersubjective relations by virtue of the affective re-creation of participants' existential plexuses, this can only transpire *in situ* and in the framework of particular group or communitarian contexts that make the emergence of this form of dialogue viable. Psychopoetics has no *essential* aspects (no essence that determines *a priori* the psychopoetic condition of a conversation). This feature does not impede, however, recognizing the relatively sustained appearance of a *critical* vocation in psychopoetic dialogue, of a more-or-less permanent, implicit, or explicit, and scathing questioning of established cultural, ideological, or political values.

Psychopoetics does not transpire in what is strictly *said* in interlocution (that is, in the properly textual or discursive terrain), nor does it occur exclusively in individual subjectivity as mere lived experience. Psychopoetics happens, precisely, in the dynamic, complex framework of relations that the interlocutors promote with the surroundings, a network of relations that includes material objects and conditions, interactive processes, and the production of diverse subjectivities which in that instant engage with the expressive reinvention in the space of the verbal exchange itself. Varied motivations; personal styles in play; shared moods; values, criteria, traditions, experiences, images, tastes, expectations, and memories that circulate *agitatedly* in that *free-dialogue* which disrupts the stability of the exchange to open the way to the creative energy of fiction and of discovery.

Psychopoetics presupposes not only the productive moment but also the *attitudinal* moment of interlocution. It is the process that includes and relates, on the one hand, the creative verbal elaboration of an approach and, on the other, the set of assumptions that bring about that which is expressed in the person or group of people that listen and look on as interlocutors of the encounter at that instant. The *psychopoetic relief* of that which is expressed thus provokes the participation of relatively sensitized subjects who attend, receive, reactivate, and re-articulate those expressions – always *in situ* – and reorient them *differentially* towards a (not imperative) continuity of *poetising* itself. Therefore, those who listen are already participating in the active re-elaboration (re-creation) of that which is said. Here I refer to that tendency which is prone to the inventive play in speech that potentiates, in effect, an *aesthetic* condition in the specific situational context because it involves unsuspected initiatives of the transformation of senses.

But we must emphasize, as well, that psychopoetics necessarily separates itself from an exegetical or hermeneutic attitude in its realization. It seeks neither to explain nor interpret what is said in order to choose a *correct meaning* of what is expressed. Clearly, it does not seek to *analyse* what is said; indeed, quite the opposite: all explicative, interpretative, or analytical exigency in interlocution (though relatively inevitable) simultaneously conditions and impedes, in one way or another, the deployment of psychopoetics. The idea is not to follow the *unfurling of language* but to escape from it; that is, to turn towards the productive *furling* of subjectivity; to brandish imaginative invention in speech that leads to immediate *revelations* of alternate worlds. The expressions of psychopoetic dialogue establish in their heterodoxy diverse ruptures and transformations of the prescriptive codes of speech, but find *pertinent* senses in the specific situational *coordinates* in which its realization occurs. The interlocutors immersed in psychopoetic dynamics put into play certain predispositions that are favourable to the creative; that suppose a certain "aesthetic optimism",[45] but do not therefore renounce the eventual exercise of *critique*.

It is due to the foregoing that the psychopoetic mood in dialogue distances itself from that interlocution marked by interventive goals and associated with codifications, schemes, and procedures of adaptation and normalization of life, in order to approach the *real* negation of social precepts and prescriptions in an exchange less concerned with *communicative order-word* (as the transmission of clear, complete messages) and more with the ever-renewed *initiatory act* of acceding to those mysterious, personal, amusing, unpredictable, and adventurous journeys of the word (fleeting events) through the intersubjective worlds of shared existence.

Notes

1 See: Lledó, E. (1961) *El concepto de "poiesis" en la filosofía griega.* Madrid: CSIC.
2 See also: Pájaro, C. (2004) Poiesis y poesía. De Homero a los sofistas. *Eidos* (2) 8–32.
3 Lledó, E. *El concepto de "poiesis" en la filosofía griega.* Ed. cit. p. 41.
4 See philosophical fragment I in: García-Bacca, J. (Selec.) (1944, 1980) *Los presocráticos.* Mexico: FCE, 2004, p. 239.
5 Pájaro, C. Poiesis y poesía. De Homero a los sofistas. Ed. cit. p. 18.
6 See also fragments 30, 53, 73, 111, and 112 from Heraclitus for their relation with the notion of *poiesis* and the verb *poien*, as well as the commentaries by Lledó and García-Bacca in this regard (*Los presocráticos.* Ed. cit. pp. 239–274; and Lledó, E. (n1) pp. 18–26).
7 See Carlos Julio Pájaro's analysis of the poetic *enthusiasmós* of Democritus in: Pájaro, C. Poiesis y poesía. De Homero a los sofistas. Ed. cit. pp. 24–28, especially the analysis of philosophical fragment 18 attributed to Democritus, also recovered by García-Bacca in his selection of texts in *Los presocráticos.* Ed. cit. p. 353.
8 Lledó, E. *El concepto de "poiesis" en la filosofía griega.* Ed. cit. p. 44.
9 Idem, pp. 46–51.
10 See the complex relation between *téchne* and *poiesis* according to Lledó's exhaustive analysis ((n1) pp. 58–63). See also Pájaro's reflection on Gorgias and poetic creation as *téchne* ((n2) pp. 28–32).
11 Plato (1931) *Diàlegs.* Barcelona: Fundació Bernat Metge. 18 Vols. 2000. *Fedre* 244 e (Vol. IX, p. 72); 245 a (p. 73). See also Lledó, E. (n1) pp. 72–74.
12 Idem, p. 74.
13 Guill, B. (1882) *Essai sur la poésie philosophique en Grèce.* Paris, p. 154 (cited by Lledó, E. (n1) p. 77).
14 Plato: *La República* Llibre X, 595 b 5 and ss. (Vol. XI, p. 97).
15 Idem, 596 c, d, e. (p. 99).
16 Idem, 600 e. (p. 106).
17 Idem, 601 b. (p. 107).
18 Lledó, E. (n1) p. 104.
19 Plato: *La República* Llibre X, 604 b. (Vol. XI, p. 113).
20 Idem, 605 b, c and ss. (p. 114–115).
21 Plato: *Leyes* Llibre III, 698 a, b.
22 Idem, 719 b 5.
23 Idem, Llibre VII, 801 d.

24 Mèlich, J. (2002) *Filosofía de la finitud.* Barcelona: Herder, p. 16.
25 Lezama, J. (1993) *La expresión americana.* Havana: Letras cubanas, p. 7.
26 Lezama, J. *La expresión americana.* Ed. cit. p. 11.
27 Idem, p. 12.
28 Idem, p. 12.
29 Idem, p. 14.
30 Diego, E. (1989) *Libro de quizás y de quién sabe.* Havana: Letras cubanas, p. 72.
31 Serres, M. *La comunicación. Hermes I.* Ed. cit. p. 297.
32 This expression is from Paul Ricoeur who uses it for *understanding*: "for a finite being, understanding [means being] transported to another life (...)" (Ricoeur, P. *El conflicto de las interpretaciones. Ensayos de hermenéutica.* Mexico: FCE, p. 11).
33 Sloterdijk, P. (2001) *Eurotaoísmo. Aportaciones a la crítica de la cinética política.* Barcelona: Seix Barral, p. 125.
34 See: Magris, C. (1993) *El anillo de Clarisse. Tradición y nihilismo en la literatura moderna.* Barcelona: Península.
35 Musil, R. (1978) *El hombre sin atributos.* Barcelona: Seix Barral, 2006. 2 Vols.
36 See: Serres, M. (1996) *La comunicación. Hermes I.* Barcelona: Anthropos.
37 See for example: Buber, M. (1923) *Yo y Tú.* Madrid: Caparrós, 1998.
38 Mèlich, J. *Filosofía de la finitud.* Ed. cit. p. 44.
39 Mèlich speaks of *technoeconomic monomythism* (Idem, p. 46).
40 For this discussion see also: Marquard, O. (2000) *Apología de lo contingente.* Valencia: Alfons el Magnànim, p. 130.
41 In these reflections I follow the work of Landa, J. (2002) *Poética.* Mexico: FCE, especially chapters III (pp. 83–130) and V (pp. 165–209).
42 Landa, J. *Poética.* Ed. cit. p. 91 (Italics added).
43 Idem, pp. 105–106.
44 Idem, pp. 119–120.
45 Idem, p. 194.

PART III

Psychopoetics: writings of imagination and amusement

7

LAS MENINAS (BY WITKIN) OR THE UNPREDICTABLE EMERGENCE OF THE POWERS OF THE SOUL[1]

I

The painter has taken a step back from the canvas. Glances over at the model with his dead eyes, one covered by a torrent of blood that runs down his face, into his beard, a serene, intriguing, almost paternal, smile emerges from his face. The arm holding the brush is inclined, ever so slightly, towards the palette, immobile for an instant between the canvas and the grey elements. His wounded hand depends on his shattered vision. Between the fine point of the brush and the abominable moment of the gaze, the spectacle directs its volume.

The painter shows a gentle, almost happy, face, which contrasts with the scene of death that surrounds him. His head is bent, somewhat rigidly, towards his shoulder, his gaze fixed upon some impossible point, but that point is ourselves, the spectators, *our* body, *our* face, *our* eyes. We might be able to intuit what the painter sees if it were possible to look at the dark canvas on which he is working, but of that all we can discern are the slats of the battered stretcher that still sustains it, in precarious equilibrium, on the verge of collapsing. That high, hidden rectangle that occupies the entire left edge of the photograph and shows us only the reverse side of the canvas represented, reconstitutes, implies, leads one to assume the invisibility, indeed, the profound, diverse unintelligibility of what the artist-cadaver is contemplating. Between the disfigured eyes of the painter and the object on which his gaze is fixed a link traverses the entire dreamlike space and carries us, irremissibly, to the terrible, fascinating

DOI: 10.4324/9781003129295-7

reality of the photograph itself, where uncertainties and figures of an incomprehensible room intersect in the tangled complex of experience. The painter takes pleasure in verifying our presence in the very place of his object, as if having once reached the scene we cannot abandon it. What seems to be happening is that, upon looking at the photograph we the spectators become trapped, in some strange way, by the painter's mocking curse and by the scene itself, into which we are unavoidably melded as if in some inevitable exchange of existences. Beside the painter we perceive what seems to be a photographic camera or projector perched atop a small circular table. This represents, in fact, a tragic reciprocity: we look upon a rectangle from which a painter-cadaver, in turn, contemplates us. Face-to-face, bloody unknown eyes, decadence, and fascination exchanged that, at the same moment, open a conspicuous web of queries: What are we doing there, in front of this scene? What play of death has trapped us in such a nightmare? What is it that the photographic camera on the small circular table captures? What is the artist painting over there in his darkened niche? Since we can see only the back of the canvas, we cannot know who we are or what we are doing there; seen or being seen?

At the instant at which the painter's dead eyes place the spectator in their field of vision, all possibility of escape disappears, we are transformed into spectator-subject, forced to assume a position that, nonetheless, seduces silently as well through the morbid proliferation of *other mysterious and sombre beings*. On the extreme right of the painting there appears, as if springing forcefully from the ground, the clear figure of a torso with an enormous head, in profile, whence protrudes a prominent, brilliant, erect tongue. Then, in the area of the torso we see two great holes that, *cum* breasts extirpated by a mad surgeon's scalpel, obscure the giant's chest like two swirls of gnawed meat. The figure somehow evokes the personages in Picasso's *Guernica*, a deformed, innocent being, a victim of inexplicable horror, a man imploring the end of a bombardment. The expression on his face mixes the enigmatic pain of tearing flesh with the steely enjoyment of mute laughter. From his left shoulder we see, like a prosthesis or malicious graft, a long outstretched arm emerging, its upper extreme an open hand with four fingers. In the extreme upper right part of the photograph, a great luminous horn emerges from the occipital area head of this giant creature (whom we might call *the man from Guernica*), like the blade of a white sickle in stark contrast to the black background, achieving a balance or equilibrium with the oblong form of the phallic tongue that rises up, on the other side, from the figure's mouth and almost touches the ceiling of the salon. The one open eye of the head, clearly delineated in black ink on the white face, reveals a prideful, animal-like, gesture as in the rictus of an irreconcilable discussion. From that same eye, projecting towards the nose and forehead, run three dotted lines like straight tears of blood that close its facial vertigo with discrete touches, never separating from the face that contains them. The eerie presence of this torso with its gigantic head produces a flow of light that spills copiously over both the surface of the painter-cadaver's canvas (one invisible to us) and the volume that the canvas might represent (that is, in the painter's study, this salon, this sinister room where he has set up his morbid easel).

As our gaze crosses the room from right to left, the light emanating from the just-described torso (its luminous nucleus seemingly in the mutilated breasts) leads the spectator-subject, at one and the same time, towards the painter and his model, towards the canvas, and this same light comes to illuminate the painter himself (situated at the extreme left of the photo), making him visible, despite his heavy black tunic, and though almost concealed in the small niche where he paints with his fine brush, palette in hand. This light produces a balance, from the opposite extreme of the image, with the painter-cadaver's invisible canvas, but simultaneously floods the scene, envelops the figures and spectator-subjects alike, and carries them, under some strange spell, towards the (inexistent) place where we come to form part of that world.

Now, right in front of the spectator-subjects – ourselves – on the background wall of the piece, the photographer captures a series of –incomplete – paintings from Velázquez' opus: on the left, *The triumph of Bacchus* or *The drunkards*, where the god of wine in far-off joy seems to peer out at us diffusely from his shared banquet; in the centre, the *Coronation of the Virgin*, the visage of María's pious rostrum barely discernible, her right hand resting on her heart, the white dove of the Holy Spirit flying glimmeringly over her head; and on the right *Apollo in the forge of Vulcan*, where the god of fire himself is visible, startled, as two of his cyclopes receive the visit of Apollo, who reveals the adultery of his beloved Venus with Mars.

All those canvases hanging in the background glow with singular resplendence. Inside their luminous frames appear diverse human figures against black backgrounds; at various points one can discern flashes of light, like distant bolts of lightning flashing against the night sky. Might these not be paintings at all but, rather, mirrors? Might that which the photographer records in the paintings in the background be nothing more than inescapable mirrors reflecting, precisely, that which we are in the moment we attend this encounter? Are we not perhaps Bacchus, triumphant for the ephemeral felicity of the drunkards who laugh and play with life? Or are we María, sublime mercy, receiving the crown of sanctity? Or perhaps we are the old god who must accept the bitterness of lost love?

None of the figures in the photo are looking at the paintings-mirrors in the back, nor is the painter or the mutilated giant, no one. The other figures in the image are turned more-or-less towards what must be occurring in front of them – towards the inexistent salon we inhabit, towards that balcony of light where their gazes see those who look at them, not in the direction of that sombre cavity into which the room where their images were captured closes in upon itself. Clearly, some of the heads appear in profile, but not one turned sufficiently to perceive the background of the piece with its high, desolate paintings-mirrors, glittering rectangles that seem to contain the most important moments of life and of the history of the world and culture (life shared with the joys of wine, celestial advent of compassion, bitter instant of broken love). We must recognize that this indifference finds its equal in their own. The paintings-mirrors, in truth, reflect nothing of all the things that exist in the space they occupy, not the painter with his back to them, not the figures in the centre of the studio. In their clear profundity they do not see the visible.

> In Dutch painting – Michel Foucault writes – it was traditional for mirrors to play a duplicating role: they repeated the original contents of the picture, only inside an unreal, modified, contracted, concave space. One saw in them the same things as one saw in the first instance of the painting, but decomposed and recomposed according to a different law.[2]

But in this photo, the paintings-mirrors proclaim something quite different, something crucial, from the lofty heights where they hang. Instead of turning towards the visible objects, they traverse (fly over) the whole field of representation, disregarding what they might capture – and reflect – there while restoring visibility to that which remains beyond any gaze. What they reflect is plurality, the heterogeneity of all that which the figures in the photograph will be forced to contemplate if they were to direct their gaze forward: it is, then, what one would see if the image were extended forward, descending further to enclose the figures that serve as the model for the painter. But it is also because the image stops there, showing the painter-cadaver and his sinister-studio-room, which is exterior to the image itself to the degree that it is a photograph, a rectangular fragment of lines and diverse tones of grey, white, and black, entrusted with recreating something to the eyes of all possible spectator-subjects or individuals. In the back of the room, ignored by all the figures, the surprising paintings-mirrors, illuminated by a light bulb hanging from the ceiling, make the personages that the painter-cadaver perceives (indeed, desires) sparkle (the painter in his overflowing world of imagination, in his longing to return to life); but also the figures that look upon the painter-cadaver or, at least, co-exist with him (in this vital reality that the photograph itself reveals). The paintings-mirrors ensure a metathesis, a projection of possibilities that break the space represented in the photo, and make it possible to see, in the upper part of the image, that which is invisible to the photograph but constitutes the very object of the painter-cadaver's desiring exercise; namely, the life that emerges from the image, the pulse of the nudity that becomes in-ebriated, and the love that is revealed intensely among people.

II

But perhaps it is time to learn the identity of the figures that appear as the personages that constitute the full composition of the photograph described. To the painter-cadaver's left, at a central point of the image there appears, in the role of protagonist, the figure of a girl with no legs (or perhaps only two stumps) resting (?) atop the pannier of a dress virtually bereft of cloth that exposes the wires of the garment's structure. The base of the pannier (and upon it, the legless girl) consists of a round platform joined to the floor by four small, dark wheels. On the platform, inside the wire structure of the pannier, we see dozens of black nails protruding upwards like a faquir's nailbed. The girl (or, more accurately, the torso of the girl placed on this structure) wears a kind of long-sleeved, white blouse with a strange black flower in the very centre of her chest. Serene of rostrum and with her hair pulled to one side in a ponytail adorned with small flowers, she stares out at us with an adult gaze (her eyes bearing a tenuous, shadowy fringe like a veil used as a mask) allowing an almost imperceptible, millimetric smile to escape her lips, as if she had caught us looking at the scene like some morbid voyeur with whom she is perfectly well acquainted. In her left hand, the girl holds an embroidered handkerchief, white in colour, that cascades smoothly over the wires of the pannier, its point just touching the nails in the bottom. In her right hand, she has a thick rope that descends to the neck of a large dog that lies asleep (or dead by poisoning) in the extreme lower right of the photo at the – non-existent – feet of the girl, whom we can call the Infanta Margarita.

To the girl's right and lower down (that is, in the extreme lower left of the image) lies the naked torso of a young man, handsome of face, who raises his strong arms from the floor over his head in a gesture reminiscent of the movements of a ballet dancer. The young man's torso reclines upon a fine cushion placed at the feet of the easel and, indeed, at the feet (though not visible either) of the painter-cadaver with his long black tunic that rises, precisely, from the fallen dancer's naked chest. In an instant, the young man's torso recalls the image of a statue toppled as if by catastrophe. His chest and abdomen are traversed by intermittent straight lines that seem to evoke the tracks left by the pneumatics of a heavy truck that had run over him.

On the wall in the background of the salon – the same wall where the paintings-mirrors hang on high, behind all the creatures described – a door opens, outlining a clear rectangle, brilliantly lit though the light does not spread widely into the room, opening outwards through its carved frame with the soft curve of a curtain and the shadow of a solitary stair. The rectangle that is the door is transformed into a diffuse but highly-intense area of clarity in which the light that does not enter completely, swirls before coming to rest upon itself. Against this backdrop, at once near and without limits, the silhouette of a tall, thin semi-naked man stands out. He too is shown in profile, placed on the very threshold of the room. He has a beard and long, black, straight hair (Christ? Alonso Quijano?). In one hand he holds, at the level of this waist, what seems from afar to be an arm of a pair of glasses or perhaps a crown of branches; the other touches the edge of the curtain.[3] His right foot is placed on the solitary stair, the left rests on the floor inside the room. He may be about to enter, or perhaps he limits himself to simply observing what is going on in the interior, satisfied to see without being seen. As with the paintings-mirrors in the background, no one pays him the slightest attention. Where he comes from or where he is going no one knows (does he come from the light, or is he moving towards it?). We might suppose, following the uncertain designs of life, that he has come to the room where the other figures are reunited and where the painter-cadaver works. But it could just as well be that an instant before he was in the foreground of the scene, in the invisible region that all the eyes in the photograph contemplate. Like the images perceptible in the background of the paintings-mirrors, it may be that he is an emissary of this vital space that we feel from the heart. There is, however, a difference: he is there in the flesh, emerging from outside into the threshold of the air-light (open sky, vertigo, uncertainty). He is not likely a reflection but, rather, an irruption, an event. The paintings-mirrors, by leading us to look beyond the walls of the studio to see what is happening in front of this image, make the interior and exterior oscillate in their sagittal dimension. The ambiguous visitor, one foot on the solitary stair, the body completely in profile, enters and leaves at the same time in a swaying immobility, somehow repeating, in his place, in the naked reality of his body, the micro-poetic movement of the bodies (our bodies), whose images traverse the salon, penetrate into the paintings-mirrors on the back wall, reflecting-recreating themselves in them to emerge-appear-be revealed once again as visible, renewed bodies-creatures-subjects identical to ourselves. Thus, the figures in the paintings-mirrors are rejected, but at the same time accepted, by the tall, solid stature of the semi-naked man who appears in the doorway and establishes a kind of brotherhood with them, something like a solidary, imperfect link whence springs, furtive and strange, a kind of hope.

But we must once again descend to the bottom of the photo, moving towards the foreground of the image, leaving behind the contour of the scroll we have been following. Upon contemplating the composition with care, it is possible to trace a series of imaginary lines that cross the entire ontology of the scene. Setting out from the gaze of the young Dionisius that appears in the extreme upper left of the photo, we can clearly draw a descending, sloping line towards the lower right margin of the round platform of Princess Margarita's pannier, precisely to the left hand of the fallen dancer. From there, another imaginary line, this one sloping slightly to the right, rising along the edge of the wire of the pannier, brushing the Infanta's right arm, and coming to rest on the head of the girl herself, in the small square of the white frame beside the open door. From this intermediate point, another sloped line descends, this one following the girl's left arm and then the structure of the pannier until it reaches the poisoned dog lying in the extreme lower right. And to complete this series of imaginary lines, another ascends from the dog's motionless body on the floor, obscured by shadows, towards the extreme upper right of the composition. This line culminates in the brief, uncertain space between the four-fingered hand of the giant (*man from Guernica*) and the luminous horn (or blade of the white sickle) that emerges from his head. Gazing upon this set of lines what is revealed, without doubt, is a large W that crisscrosses the entire surface of the image.

But another set of lines must also be highlighted: one running from the spot in the upper left corner of the photo where the young Bacchus appears and the place where the poisoned dog lies in the bottom right corner. The central point of this long diagonal line coincides with the lower abdomen –occult – of the Princess. Another long diagonal line can be traced between the left arm and hand of the fallen dancer in the lower left corner and the luminous horn that sprouts from the head of the giant of Guernica. This line also passes through the hidden sex of the legless girl before extending, as if in an instant of diffraction, along the entire arm that stretches upwards from the giant's shoulder. It is as if in a final, desperate gesture of battle, the dancer had thrown some terrible projectile, made of desire and the strength of his arm itself, towards the giant's body, passing through the girl's dress and (pulverized) hips to inflict that great wound-gnawing of meat on the figure's chest, before exiting through its shoulder-back towards the other extreme, provoking the rictus of pain and death etched so visibly on the creature's face. Observing these two diagonal lines together reveals a large "X" that also presides over the entire image. Thus we perceive the simultaneous existence of two sets of lines that form the letters "W" and "X". In the play of meanings produced therein, the "W" obviously pertains to Witkin, while the "X" is the unknown value of an existential equation that could pertain to any one of us.

The frieze that occupies the different planes of the photo presents – if we include the painter-cadaver – six figures. Of these, three are looking directly at those who gaze upon them (ourselves). The centre of this group is dominated by the small, legless Infanta with her shadowed eyes and ample, wire pannier with no cloth. Her rostrum is located at the very focal point of the image, approximately at two-thirds of the total height of the frame. Without doubt, this is where the principle theme of the composition resides, the essential object of the photograph. As if to prove and underscore this even more, the author includes the figure that, placed to one side and below the central personage, appears to be paying her tribute with his outstretched arms. Like some fallen angel venerating the broken-virgin, the dancer's torso lying on the floor extends its arms towards the Princess, his face framed in perfect profile at the girl's non-existent feet. To the right of the Infanta, the giant with erect tongue and ravaged chest seems to retreat from the force of her presence, as if leaning slightly backwards to allow her to advance on her round platform with its small black wheels.

Finally, three more figures: the semi-naked man in the open door in the back, the painter-cadaver on the dark, left fringe, and the poisoned dog in the lower right corner. Arranged in this way, they seem to be constituted as a kind of sinister escort of the Princess as she advances in the centre. But when seen together, and if one pays attention to the point of reference, another interesting geometric figure can be seen to form, this

one charged with a profound meaning: it is a large triangle, its base
formed by the straight line that begins at the painter-cadaver's eyes, passes
across the face of the semi-naked man in the open doorway, and culminates in the face of the giant, its sharp vortex placed on the hidden
heart of the immobile, poisoned dog lying on the floor. This large triangle
has no other purpose than to reveal to us, in all its stark beauty, the
omnipresent pubis of a naked woman (note here, the unmistakeable si-
milarity between Witkin's photograph and Courbet's painting *The origin
of the world*). If we observe this anatomy in detail, the pubic hair that
grows is on the dark wall of the background and the figure of the Princess
constitutes, integrally, the vagina that opens, mysterious and terrible,
through the empty pannier: "A dream without throat/ a slow passageway
where two bodies fit/ that are going to be inaugurated under the dawn of
the world"[4] And, once more, at the crucial point of the panorama, the
Infanta's face, revealing itself as the perfect clitoris that looks (looks at us)
without prudishness, that touches with its intense presence that most
abominable instant of desire, basking in the veneration proffered by a
fallen dancer.

> If you had a less imposing clitoris
> I would not feel your loss
> if you were more distant with more measured stubbornness
> my kidney would sing for a week
> I am as nothing you are more distant than ever before
> and walk with my pirouette and face of death
> with a bit of absence under the arms and I walk
> with water to live with my armpit that shouts
> I have only two eyes and an impassive thirst (...)[5]

Finally, what is to be found in this perfectly inaccessible place, the one
outside the image, but demanded by all the effects of the composition?
What is the spectacle, what are the rostrums reflected, first, in the pupils
of the Infanta, then in those of the painter-cadaver and of the man in
the doorway in the background and, finally, in the far-away clarity of the
paintings-mirrors? But this question doubles back upon itself: the faces
reflected in the paintings-mirrors and those that contemplate them; what
all the personages of the photograph see, are also the subjects to whose
eyes they are offered as a scene to contemplate. The image in its totality
sees a scene for which it is, in turn, a scene. Or perhaps we are not dealing
with a scene at all but, rather, with a factory. A factory, a *big generator* of

desiring production whose formidable lines of articulation involve a terrible, but beautiful, reciprocity that extends into the tangle of lights and shadows.

This brief glimpse of the image has allowed us to discover in what this spectacle we see consists (this production overflowing with meaning): ourselves. We are what is perceivable in the enigmatic gaze of the legless girl, in the amazement, the pain, and the furtive felicity of the faces and bodies that inhabit the photograph and seem to move, speak, escape, and invent another indescribable universe. Amidst all these strange faces, all these destroyed bodies, we are the most intense, the most real, the most committed of all the presences. Of all these personages/creatures/subjects, we are also the most mysterious because no one pays attention to the flash that springs upon the world from our chest and introduces itself silently through an unsuspected space. To the degree to which we are invisible, we are the strongest and closest form to all reality. And vice versa, to the same degree to which, residing outside the image, we are distant in an essential invisibility, ordered, configured, moulded by the image itself: those are the personages who mark us with their presence, who make our eyes move; it is towards us that the amorous mandate of the Infanta with her torn dress and tragic destiny is directed. It is in this situation that the gaze of the girl and the images of the paintings-mirrors are ordered and made to appear in the centre of the composition to which, ultimately, they are subjected. This centre is the infinite subjectivity capable of producing unrepeatable and diverse meanings through the multiple landscapes of existence.

In the large scroll that frames the perimeter of the studio, from the gaze of the painter-cadaver with his palette and paused hand, to the hidden heart of the Infanta, the production of subjectivity is born with great strength and is realised in its own sovereignty to be recomposed, anew, in light and shadow: the cycle imperfect and infinite. Added to this, the lines that crisscross in the profundity of the image are articulated and completed in a certain unknown region of affect, whose trajectory appears to be concentrated, again, in the girl's body, whence it is prolonged by diffraction, and then flees, with unspeakable enthusiasm, towards the clear morning of the world.

Perhaps in this photograph, as in every moment of invention in which life is manifested, so to speak, the overflowing imagination of what is seen is solidary with the imagination of he who looks – in spite of the darkness, of the inertias, of the suppressions, of the desolation. Concomitantly with the image and its forms, there emerge as well the forms of subjective fertility, extended as an offering. In the profundity that traverses the image a fiction and a kind of felicity is generated in whose eclosion an obstinate presence is signalled imperiously and everywhere: the necessary affirmation of the creative instant and of the subject that feels and exercises its expression. This same subject, with all its impurities and freedom has been incorporated, once again, and pronounces itself (despite its reiterated deaths) one of the more unpredictable potencies of the planet.

Notes

1 It was in 1966 that Michel Foucault published in French *Les Mots et les Choses. Une archéologie des sciences humaines*. In Chapter I, entitled "Les suivantes" (in Spanish, "Las Meninas"), the author develops a detailed analysis of Velázquez' well-known painting of the same name (1656) in which he reflects upon its signs and forms of *representation*. In the present text, as a humble tribute to Foucault's text, I follow his words to the letter but while analysing Joel-Peter Witkin's 1987 photograph, entitled "Las Meninas (Autorretrato según Velázquez)" (see Annex 1) and then, based on the variations and derivations there described, venture into the terrain of recognizing the inventive potential of subjectivity. The text utilized was the Spanish translation of Foucault's book (1968): Foucault, M. (1966) *Las palabras y las cosas. Una arqueología de las ciencias humanas*. Madrid: Siglo XXI, 1968, 2005, pp. 13–25. The version used for the English translation of my text is: Foucault, M. (1966) *The Order of Things. An Archaeology of the Human Sciences*. New York: Vintage Books, 1970.

2 Foucault, M. (1966) *The Order of Things. An Archaeology of the Human Sciences*. New York: Vintage Books, 1970, p. 7.

3 See: Franceschini, C.; Cecereu, L. (thesis adviser) (n/d) *Memorias olvidadas. Joel Peter Witkin. Una obra fotográfica contemporánea acerca de lo ominoso*. Thesis to obtain a Master's Degree in the Theory and History of Art. Universidad de Chile, Facultad de Artes. To probe more deeply into the analysis of Witkin's work, see as well: Ugarte, S.; Vilar, G. (thesis director) (2006) *Al otro lado del espejo. Lo abyecto en la estética fotográfica de Joel-Peter Witkin*. Doctoral Thesis, Universidad Autónoma de Barcelona, Facultad de Filosofía y Letras.

4 Fernández Larrea, R. (1989) Fragment of the poem: "Lejos" in: *Poemas para ponerse en la cabeza*. Havana: Editora Abril, p. 19.

5 Fernández Larrea, R. (1989), Fragment of the poem: "Quince centavos en el bolsillo izquierdo" in: *Poemas para ponerse en la cabeza*. Havana: Editora Abril, p. 15.

8

THE BOTTLE OF BEAUJOLAIS: A (NOT OVERLY) CRITICAL DISCOURSE ANALYSIS

To Ian Parker

Introduction

Discourse is constituted as a fundamental way of being in the world. In the avatars of human existence, things become, are interwoven and configured, interrelate and share; though the ways may be unpredictable, they are always discursive. It is through discourse that the self achieves some of its possible, or virtual, integrations. To discourse is to exist, and to exist is to discourse. The product of this process is *discourse* in all its diversity. But discoursing also entails being in relation with other discourses, opening up to other intellections of the world and in one voice tracing the sensitive specificity and irreproducible character of those who discourse. Hence, acceding to a discursive order means producing it through participant interaction, the delineation of which often anticipates unexpected outcomes. The discursive order constantly reinvents itself through the participation of those who speak; discourse means, as well, making things flow in certain senses while we simultaneously flow with the things through the world, and in this movement, inhabit and sense it in a certain way.[1]

In his 1992 text, *Discourse Dynamics: Critical Analysis for Social and Individual Psychology*, Ian Parker proposes – something akin to – a specific procedure or method of critical discourse analysis, one that could lead to a study of the dynamics, tensions and forms of reproduction of discourses

DOI: 10.4324/9781003129295-8

through their linkages with the transformation of the world and the subjectivities entailed.[2] Parker holds that discourses susceptible to analysis are only spoken interactions or previously-given written forms, but those constituted as *texts*, understood as "delimited tissues of meaning reproduced in any form".[3] Here, any object comprehended in some way in terms of a specific interweaving of significations and meanings can be analysed as a textual form, including traffic lights, fashion or architecture (in fact, some years later, Parker presented a critical-discursive analysis of a children's toothpaste, entitled "Punch and Judy", where he reflects on the packaging, physical features and, of course, the written instructions, all in relation to its articulation with the social worlds involved).[4] Parker's proposal elaborates a set of ten criteria required to develop such analyses, then derives from each one distinct concrete steps for its realization. Studies of this kind must expose the contradictions and problems of the political dimension (institutions, power, ideology) of the objects of the discourse analyzed. The present work (which adopts Parker's critical proposal, though perhaps in a heterodox, free manner) proposes analyzing a **bottle of Beaujolais** to reveal not only its political, but also − if conceivable − its *poetic* reality.

Analysis

Primer criterion: a discourse is realized in texts

Analytical step number 1: express the object of study in written language; that is, describe it in words, transform it to text

It is no easy thing to transform a bottle of Beaujolais into written language, especially when the analyst is − simultaneously − savouring its contents. But with the greatest rigour possible, I shall assay to express this magnificent product in words, well-aware, obviously, that any similar *transcription* will of necessity be distinct from what another subject would compose, such as the producer, publicist, oenologist, or a musician. Also, the description offered actually changes from moment-to-moment, for a recently-uncorked bottle of Beaujolais is not the same once its rich contents has been imbibed − alone or accompanied − amidst diverse joys and/or sorrows depending, as well, on what people or animals are present.

What I can affirm, to begin, is that my Beaujolais is in a 30-centimetre tall, green-hued bottle with a capacity for 750 millilitres of wine. Amiable and elegant to the eye, it has the traditional burgundy form. The wine inside appears as a very dark, strong liquid that, held against the light, turns intensely red with mysterious transparencies. The wrapping around its mouth is light brown with a tenuous metallic tonality. In the centre, one perceives a small gold seal showing a deer's head surrounded by vines. Under a straight line at the base of the wrapping we read in gold-lettering *–no less –* the name *ALBERT BICHOT*, then, where the body of the bottle begins, a second modest label, beige, that reads *RECOLTE* in gold, slightly-curved lettering, and just below that, but in black, the year *2009*, over a fine gold point. Next comes the main label, covering much of the body of the bottle. It is 12 centimetres wide by 9 centimetres high with a beige background, made of paper with a slightly roughened texture, perhaps simulating the softness of tanned leather. It has a square drawn with a fine line of white ink, while at its base there is a thin black fringe (that blends somewhat with the colour of the wine). There, in the centre, but in white ink, appears the name *ALBERT BICHOT*, separated by the re-appearance of the small gold, deer's head seal, still garlanded by vines. The upper-middle area of this label shows the Bichot family's coat-of-arms: a royal blue oval containing, in miniature in white ink, three pine trees above the silhouette of a deer with no antlers. Above the blue oval one observes a nine-pointed gold crown and, flanking the oval and crown, two svelte mastiffs (gold-coloured dogs that could boast extraordinary strength, loyalty and courage as guardians of property capable of fending off fierce beasts) in aggressive stances but their heads looking backwards, as if to protect the oval and crown on the coat-of-arms. All this is etched upon a cone-shaped gold base that in terms of architectural structure brings to mind the roof of a pagoda. On the left of the shield we read in small letters, *Depuis*; on the right, *1831*, and beneath, *PRODUIT DE FRANCE*. Next, in the very centre of the label, in large, black capital letters printed with a shadowing technique, *BEAUJOLAIS*, and under that, but in small letters, *Appellation d'origine controlee*. Further below, in larger letters is the legend *Sélection Parcellaire*, followed by a short gold line and, lower still, in small black letters, the message: *Elevé et mis in bouteille par Albert Bichot a Beaune, Bourgogne, France.* Two more details: first, at the extreme lower left of the main label, the legend in grey, *12,5% vol.*; and at the extreme lower right, also in grey, *75 cl*; second: on the left side in very small grey letters written vertically, one reads *Contient sulphites-contains sulphites-Enthält Sulphite-Indeholder Sulfitter*. Also written in vertical lines on the right, but in letters so small and grey as to be almost imperceptible, the message: *La consommation de boissons alcoolisées pendant la grossesse, meme en faible quantité, peut avoir des conséquences graves sur la santé d l'enfant.*

Analytical step number 2: explore the connotations of the text through a form of free association (best performed when accompanied)

The first time I heard the word *Beaujolais* was in 1985 when, as a youth, I discovered an LP by The Alan Parsons Project called *Stereotomy*, whose thin cardboard cover showed, beside an illustration that may have been an image from an old Rorschach test, the lyrics of the songs printed in white. There, in song 2, "Side A", I read "Beaujolais", translated into Spanish for a certain sector of the Latin American music market as *Vino francés* (*i.e.*, French wine). I didn't know (and didn't much care) – until later in life – what this oh so French, oh so strange, word meant; after all, what could I have known of gamay grapes or the Beaujeu Castle? I just liked dancing to the chords:

> No clock beside my bed
> Don't try to wake me
> No phone upon my wall
> Who's going to call?
> No knock upon my door
> No news to shake me
> Nights like the one before
> I can't take no more

It must have been life with its uncertainty-filled travels, plus the garden of delicacies, the pensive harlequin and the pains that are erased but reemerge like a landscape or ship that sails away, that would lead me to discover the wine I am drinking, that nourishes me and makes me strong to bear the onslaughts of existence. And it must have been the big city that grew from my feet up to the planets, with its nocturnal avenues and yellow-lit streets, and the endearing cold, that led me to the profound understanding of my steps and to unceasingly hop around the house:

> Beaujolais goes straight to my head
> Beaujolais puts me to shame
> And I don't know why I'm in this place or how I came
> Beaujolais and I go crazy
> Beaujolais I can't explain
> But it helps me to forget the past and ease the pain

Precisely because there are so many lonely hearts in the real world, the bottle of Beaujolais transforms itself into George Méliés' rocket that since 1902, like some gigantic cannonball, is shot out and climbs to the moon, while I travel inside that enormous ball seeing in the stars the rostrum of sweetness before landing abruptly on a crying face, then trapped by lunatics, against whom I rebel and struggle until I escape and return to Paris full of glory to receive a huge medal. Then we all dance, everyone full of joy:

> One race that I can't win
> With an alter ego
> One chance to sink or swim
> What am I to do?

The bottle of Beaujolais contains an *aleph* and cosmos that open up and concentrate at a point of convergences. As we savour the wine we also imbibe the entire universe, geographies, mysteries, unexpected turns of intimacy, the fury of the astronomer, and magic, late-evening fields and stories of spoils and envies of family businesses, but also the dawning of a century and happy bodies having loved, the hopes of southern France, the deep gaze of the unmentionable woman, and the music that makes us dance at night, and the luck of setting out in search of more adventures with the Lunarians or perhaps encountering the sea.

If someone asked me, I would reply that the bottle of wine is an ever-luminous pleat that resists and impedes diverse unfoldings of power, for each time my cup is filled with that flash of blood, power disappears, though no one knows anything, and the Beaujolais becomes a zone of meaning that articulates the creation of a new soul. Might I also become such a serious man of joyous character, perhaps in a cup of wine *on a festive night when the stars shall fall from the sky and I shall drink the thunder in great swigs and shall laugh out loud with the rays in my heart* and perhaps my soul is liquid, guilty, of intense (bluish) red colour, inhabiting an average body perhaps tending towards robustness, and perhaps an aroma of blueberries cherries raspberries and gooseberries begins to hover as if to say that (if I drink this wine) I will be a fruity man, but one elegant, or only another stranger in the world, lover of wild roses who dances while growing old in oaken casks:

> Beaujolais goes straight to my head
> Beaujolais' the one to blame

And I don't know why I'm in this place or how I came
Beaujolais I can't complain
Cause it helps me to forget the past and ease the pain.

Second criterion: a discourse on objects

Analytical step number 3: detail (define) systematically the objects that appear in the text

In the bottle of Beaujolais, one can appreciate (as the cups keep coming) at least 21 *objects* (units of logic or names) that allow us to foresee and understand the kinds of worlds that the bottle presupposes and re-creates each time it is read or that its contents are consumed or shared in life.

The first object to appear, imposing its presence through its very materiality, is the **burgundy bottle** itself; the dark green-coloured recipient with its graceful, elegantly-curved form and 750-millilitre capacity for wine (or some other liquid). Unlike its more widely-used cousin, the broader-shouldered Burdeos-style bottle, this *botella borgoñesa* is un-questionably more feminine, reminiscent of Duke Ellington's sophisti-cated lady, attired in an elegant evening gown.

The next object is the contents, the **red wine** inside the bottle of Beaujolais that might soberly be defined as the "beverage produced by the complete or partial alcoholic fermentation of fresh grapes or must. Its degree of alcohol content may not fall below 9° except in special cases".[5] Perceived more profoundly, however it could perhaps be defined as *líquida alma de mujer* or *relámpago de sangre* (the liquid soul of woman or blood lightning).

The next element to catch our attention is the **wrapping around the mouth of the bottle**, an accoutrement of specially-made paper that protects the mouth while it remains corked, and that almost always bears the em-blem of the wine-making house. What stands out here is the **seal with the deer's head surrounded by vines**, shown in gold colour over the light brown background and tenuous metallic tonality that distinguishes the material that embraces the neck of the bottle; the seal that is the official emblem of these winemakers that seeks to inspire *tradition, seriousness, elegance*.

After that, the eye catches the important legend, **Albert Bichot**, which seems to constitute itself as the backdrop and most consistent logic upon which the entire process of producing the bottle of Beaujolais is based.

At this point, another key object attracts one's attention: the bottle's **main label**, its "letter of presentation" that suggests a promise at once beautiful, simple and elegant, yet never boastful, pompous or filled with fanfare.

Then there is the **secondary label**, added to complement the "letter of presentation": a second piece of paper, an aerodynamic figure strategically placed between the *chest* and *neck* of the bottle that bears fundamental information: *Recolte 2009* (2009 harvest).

The next object that stands out is nothing less than the **Bichot family's coat-of-arms**, the golden jewel from the main label that combines the symbolism of a lineage of aristocratic ascendance while also underscoring the family's years of experience and dedication to winemaking: *Depuis 1831* (since 1831).

The next element we would highlight is the one that seems to re-present the very nucleus, the essence, that integrates the heterogeneity of the reality just described: the simple, isolated word **Beaujolais**, solemnly, even radiantly placed at the very focal point of the main label whence it projects nobility, gallantry, elegant serenity and endearing affection (I adore this object especially; so much, indeed, that it merits another long sip of wine with an international *salute* to all my friends).

After that, several objects parade before my eyes to, quite discretely, reinforce, in terms of context, the affective nucleus constituted by the *Beaujolais*. There is the legend that reads **produit de France**: national vindication, a nation's lifeblood, ostentation of pleasure; followed immediately by a second line: **appellation d'origine controlée** (denomination of origin), the discrete announcement that *this* wine – and *only* this wine – comes from, and was elaborated in, that specific place of origin. Next we read: **sélection parcellaire**, suggesting that the wine is produced by a special, unique technique using grapes from a particular, geographically well-delimited area. Then we read: **élevé et mis in bouteille par Albert Bichot to Beaune, Bourgogne, France** (elaborated and bottled by Albert Bichot in Beaune, Burgundy, France) that further emphasizes the strict quality control applied when producing this special wine.

Further down, finally, we can appreciate another series of objects, but these are of a more informative, perhaps technical, character that reflect the processes involved in the biopolitical regulation of wine consumption: **12,5% vol.**: the degree of alcohol content of the beverage to be savoured; **75 cl**: the amount of liquid that the bottle holds; **Sulphites**: mineral or organic salts from sulphurous acid that are added to the wine at a strategic moment to slow down the fermentation process and eliminate micro-organisms; **Consommation de boissons alcoolisées** (consumption of alcoholic beverages): the warning that one should consume wine with moderation but, of course, this after one has already acquired and – likely – tasted the wine inside the bottle of Beaujolais; *La grossesse* (pregnancy): a condition that may well be the result of a fertile man and ovulating woman drinking a bottle of Beaujolais until they get so carried away by erotic enthusiasm that they forget to take care to use some method of birth control; and **Faible quantité** (small amount): the great hypocrisy, I mean, after all, you open the bottle of Beaujolais because you want to drink all the wine inside. On this point, we find that producers, merchandisers and consumers all agree, *vive la France*. Then a grim warning: **Consequences graves** that no one wants to suffer but that may come from drinking too much red wine from the bottle of Beaujolais. And, finally, **Santé de l'enfant** (children's health), but who the hell is thinking of kids' wellbeing as they imbibe fine wine from the bottle we're analysing.

Of course, other objects could be added or perhaps associated with these observations, depending on the circumstances of the get-together or the precise setting; no doubt, they would lead to elaborating certain *ethno-epistemic-affective* combinations[6] or specific networks, diverse socio-material and emotional weavings. These elements might include, for example, the corkscrew, the fruit perched on the blue tablecloth, the evening shadows on the windows, the eyes of the woman you adore, an affectionate pooch, tobacco smoke, aromatic, recently-prepared food, remembrances of Paris, music, bitter memories or books.

Analytical step number 4: allude to the styles or forms of speaking (in turn) as objects of study or discourses

In this bottle of Beaujolais there co-exist different styles or distinct forms of speaking or discourses that when articulated in a specific and harmonious manner produce an interweaving of cultural and symbolic identities that strongly impacts how we conceive the worlds on the bottle itself but, above all, how one may savour the wine while imbibing it. What parade before my eyes in this case are, basically, three forms or styles of speech or discourse:

1. *An aristocratic form or style, traditional French elegance reflecting discrete opulence with a subtle hint of arrogance.*
    This discourse is present in the set of elements that define, then emphasize, the supposed social category, wealth, tradition, lineage and prestige of the bottle of Beaujolais. It is mostly concentrated in the upper part of the main label. I'm referring to the discrete gold lettering that says *Depuis 1831*; the elegant

message *Produit de France*; the coat-of-arms upon its royal blue oval; the far-away pine trees, the deer, and, of course, the gold-coloured mastiffs alertly standing guard over this exalted symbol carefully place right beside the nine-pointed crown. Added to this, we find the main legend from the label repeated in larger, shadowy black letters. A presence that definitively, un-questionably, yet baldly, states *BEAUJOLAIS*. And, of course, the two legends that identify *Albert Bichot* – one on the wrapping around the mouth of the bottle, the other at the base of the main label – alluding so clearly to the prosperous *Maison* with high-lights in gold and white accompanied by the discrete emblem of the deer's head surrounded by vines.

2. *A professional form or style of quality control in European winemaking.*
    We see this speech form, or discursive style, with great clarity in the several messages alluding to the rigours of process and the controls imposed on wine production, including the following elements: the legend on the second label, strategically placed between the bottle's *chest* and *neck*, which states: *Recolte 2009*. I associate this with the messages on the main label that say: *Apellation d'origine controlée*; *Sélection parcellaire* (alluding to the technique of selecting grapes from a specific, delimited area) and *Élevé et mis en bouteille par Albert Bichot a Beaune, Bourgogne, France*.

3. *A technical-scientific form or style inspired in biopolitics.*
    This third form or style of speech or discourse appears in the data and messages carefully placed at discrete – almost occult – points of the main label. In this sense, we find the wine's alcohol content – 12,5% *vol* – the volume of liquid or capacity of the bottle – 75*cl* – the warning message – in four languages, no less, French, English, German, and Danish – that the wine contains sulphites and a second warning – only in French – that "con-suming alcoholic drinks while pregnant, even in small amounts, can have serious consequences for the child's health".

Third criterion: a discourse contains subjects

Analytical step number 5: identify the subjects present in the text

Without doubt, the first subject present in the text (though perhaps only *indirectly*) and the appearance (to me as analyst) of the bottle of Beaujolais,

could be none other than **Mr. Bernard Bichot**, that great-grandson of a
Corbeton nobleman, founder of the *House of Bichot's* family business in
Monthélie around 1831; in reality, the man who made the whole en-
terprise and history possible (what would my life be without him!). Then
our eyes are drawn to the name **Hippolyte Bichot**, Bernard's son, pur-
chaser of the original vineyards in Volnay (so important), then **Albert
Bichot I**, Bernard's grandson, who in the late 19th century led the family
business in a new direction, eventually establishing it in central Beaune
around 1912. The next figure to come to mind is **Albert Bichot II** (born
1900), a traveller to North America, Asia and Oceania, and promotor and
pioneer of international trade in wines produced by the Bichot family. It
was he who – among other exploits – began to export wine to North
America once Prohibition, which banned imports of alcohol, was re-
pealed. Next, I read **Albert Bichot II's children** (Albert, Bernard, Jean
Marc, Benigna), heirs of the family's entrepreneurial experience in the
mid-20th century, when construction began on a cavernous building
designed to age and bottle the wine, and on new installations for wine
production. This brings us to another key figure, **Alberic Bichot**, wine-
maker and producer *par excellence* who came into this world in 1964 and,
after exploring far-off geographies around the planet, returned home to
become the General Director of the *House of Albert Bichot* (a position he
still holds as I pen these lines). Alberic's clearly French countenance reveals a figure we can only describe as a 'jolly good fellow'. But I must
move, immediately, to the next group of subjects: *the women, wives and/
or mothers* and the contributions, efforts and actions of their sex and
placentas (who knows how much joy or sadness, suffering or hope) in
giving birth to, and raising, this pleiad of wine-producers. For reasons
beyond my comprehension, they are not given a place of honour in the
official history of the *House of Albert Bichot* (though the coat-of-arms does
vindicate the figure of a *deer*). As no details of their lives are revealed, who
knows what feminine mysteries might lie behind this bottle of Beaujolais.
In contrast, I find myself perfectly able to identify with the *company's
team of producers* (described on its website as the *art* and *talent* behind the
production process, and including winemakers, supervisors, oenologists,
agronomists, managers, *sumelliers*, field supervisors, scientists, researchers
and promoters of culture). Now this group has some really interesting
names, like Alain Serveau, Mateo Mangenot, Christophe Chauvel,
Martial Beauvais, Cyril Jacquelin, Yves Decosne. Of course, I can readily
identify, as well, with the groups of *fieldworkers* who perform the
most extenuating manual labour in winemaking culture; a collective of
perhaps 100 folks (for a company with annual operations valued around

45.5 million Euros); another group of subjects that never receives its due, but one with no interesting names. Who knows, once again, what histories of these simple folk lie behind this bottle of Beaujolais. And the same could be said of the **international merchandizers and distributors**, quite anonymous they, but devoted to generating quite handsome profits. I could, by way of example, mention the people who run *Bodegas la Negrita*, a company that (as I write these lines) is busily commercializing and distributing the *Albert Bichot* trademark in México. Finally, just one figure more: someone as crucial for the text I am writing and for all possible analyses of the discourse that I might draft in this case; I refer to **the woman who gave me the bottle of Beaujolais**; such an enchanting soul who shares with me immeasurable quantities of alcohol but does not suffer fools lightly. She, whose name is "made of the sound of flying doves"[7] is the definitive condition for the appearance of that bottle before my eyes and the person mainly responsible for the pleasure that similar wines produce upon my palate, of the corporal dispositions they provoke, and of the dreams they unleash. Under what mystery of universal concatenation and destiny of the world does it become possible to wander along the archway that runs from the mercantile wiliness of that descendant of the Burgundian nobility, to the hands and gaze of the woman I love. Might life itself carry the incomprehensible pulse of that eternal return that resonates in the word? As Borges expressed it in his well-known verses:

> *Los ponientes y las generaciones (…).*
> *El ojo descifrando la tiniebla.*
> *El amor de los lobos en el alba.*
> *La palabra. El hexámetro. El espejo (…).*
> *Las manzanas de oro de las islas.*
> *Los pasos del errante laberinto (…).*
> *La moneda en la boca del que ha muerto (…).*
> *la sombra de las cruces en la tierra (…).*
> *Los rastros de las largas migraciones.*
> *La conquista de reinos por la espada.*
> *La brújula incesante. El mar abierto (…).*
> *La escrupulosa línea del calígrafo.*
> *El rostro del suicida en el espejo (…).*
> *Las formas de la nube en el desierto (…).*
> *Cada remordimiento y cada lágrima.*
> *Se precisaron todas esas cosas*
> *Para que nuestras manos se encontraran.*[8]

The sunsets and generations (...).
The eye deciphering the dark.
The love of wolves at dawn.
The word. The hexameter. The mirror (...).
The golden apples on the islands.
The steps in the wandering labyrinth (...).
The coin in the dead man's mouth (...).
The shadow of the crosses over the earth (...).
The footprints of long migrations.
The conquest of kingdoms by the sword.
The relentless compass. The open sea (...).
The calligrapher's meticulous line.
The face of the suicidal one in the mirror (...).
The shapes of a cloud in the desert (...).
Each regret and each tear.
All those things were necessary
For our hands to meet.

Analytical step number 6: reconstruct (speculatively) what the subjects involved in the text would have to say in the context of rules presupposed by the text itself

At an impossible reunion, several members of the Bichot family are chatting, accompanied by other subjects implicated in the appearance of the bottle of Beaujolais before me. The bottle itself is perched atop a small coffee table in view of all those present and myself. Striving to perform my function of analyst, I sit discretely in a corner of the living room, raptly listening to the group's conversation and busily scribbling notes:

– "Remember, I was the one who began to travel in earnest!" –stated Albert Bichot II – "and to spread the product around the world; the decision to take it to America, that country where there'd be money for everything... and money is everything... that's what was so clever, the door that opens..."
– "Well, I would have liked to keep traveling the world" – interrupts Alberic Bichot, almost totally bald in his blue-grey shirt and black jacket – "and exploring without having to worry about running the family business... but all of you have called me back... and here I am... forced to take control of everything, like directing an orchestra" – and as he said that everyone noted his stunned rostrum –

"I'm not complaining, mind you, but you've got to understand that I'm the present, I'm the one who faces today's challenges, like shifting us to ecological agriculture in our *Cote d' Or* vineyards; or finding and adapting to new markets and, you know, the whole issue of promoting and disseminating wines from the region…"

Bernard Bichot, garbed in a rather antiquated, yet still elegant, brown suit, felt hat and fine tie, is seated like a patriarch, his hands resting on the gold grip of his cane. Though surely loath to admit it, and though keeping his lips arched in a petulant gesture, I could intuit that, out of some strange egoism, he felt a deep sense of contentment with his legacy, beyond family squabbles and secrets. And at that instant he intervened, his voice metallic, his speech paused:

– "My spirit and smile lie behind this bottle of Beaujolais and I am, pardon the expression, the shadow that lit the path… if it hadn't been for that trading house in Monthélie, you, my progeny, would never have achieved what you enjoy today"…

His son, Hippolyte, replies immediately with an educated gesture, looking at the rest:

– "Father… I've always respected you, as you well know, but I have to say that without those first vineyards in Volnay, and their strategic location, we never would've progressed beyond the condition of small-scale merchants…"

With deliberate promptness, a rather anonymous woman (of unknown name) who had been whispering with another in a dimly-lit corner of the room, raises her voice to say:

– "That's all well and good, but those of us who have organized daily life, meals, children, correct manners, and the sex you enjoy so much! (that's right, Alberic! there you have me fornicating with you like a bitch every time you wanted – she says, her delicate hands atwitch – and who have never complained, giving birth to one and all, well, that's *us*! Why don't you mention *us*? Why doesn't the company ever mention *us*? What would become of the *maison* without *us*? And, for that matter, what would become of you without *us*? We don't wonder where our men are but, rather, where *our names* are?... and that's doesn't even include any questioning of the whole issue of finances!"

— "I agree" – another voice breaks in – "what about the manual labors of producing in the vineyards in the winery, and in the basements, that's the work we do..."

— "Well said!" – concurs the booming voice of Alain Serveau (a rather ugly fellow, though with a pleasant smile, wearing a dark blue jacket, a checkered handkerchief in the pocket) – "visiting wine-producing regions, controlling production techniques, imbuing each wine with its own particular *style*..."

— "And what about all the years of training to become an oenologist!" – exclaims Christophe Chauvel, a man of distracted gaze, short-cropped hair and half-grown beard, in shirtsleeves – "and then practicing ecological agriculture... that's no small thing."

— "Nor is evaluating the potential of each harvest, or selecting the wood for the casks" – chimes in Cyril Jacqueline, the youngest of all, yet sporting a dense beard and deep, dark eyes, still wearing his work apron; then adding in an ironic tone: "We're the true *art and talent* of the bottle of Beaujolais!", and the room echoes with gales of laughter.

— "We'll see about that!" – harrumphs Albert Bichot I, gesturing in desperation – "if it is of merit that we are to speak, may I remind you that the definitive entrepreneurial push, well, that came from me! For I knew how to take advantage of the phylloxera crisis and I succeeded in purchasing those small wineries in Burgundy; in fact, thanks to that growth we were able to leave the installations in Meursault and set up shop in Beaune, in the San Nicolás neighborhood... so if our bottle of Beaujolais has come so far... the credit is mine."

— "We've inherited the company and it's done well by us" – Jean Marc Bichot points out, speaking in plural to include his brothers – "we've fulfilled our duty by developing it; after all, wasn't it us who took charge of constructing the new aging and bottling plant and the new warehouse?... but please, our discussions must never leave this room; no one needs to learn of these personal ambitions, these frustrated lives, the bitterness..."

— "No doubt" – adds Alberic, with a certain solemnity in his expression, assuming his role as the company's General Director – "what's important is that we have achieved many great things and benefited many people; we're true patrons of culture; we sponsor the prize for literature awarded each September in the *Clos de Vougeot*;[9] we associate with the Writers' Club of Burgundy; support the festival of "music and wine"; perform do philanthropic works (remember the wines auctioned for charity every November); provide scholarships to young artists with talent; support the international festival of *suspense* cinema in Beaune and, of course, we foment the culinary life of Burgundy!...

- "Oh, the beef stew!" – interrupts vehemently old Bernard, overcome by a sudden wave of melancholy and a desire to come back to life.
- "The pleasures of the table and the lifestyle" – concludes Alberic – "after six generations there is no more important moment for our wine than the present..."

At that moment, three young winery workers enter (two men and a woman). One of them asks:

- "*Monsieur* Alberic, we've finished repairing the plow and brought the fertilizer; any other orders?"
- "Not for now" – responds the General Director – "*merci*, tomorrow return to your normal activities..."
- "*Oui monsieur*".

It is then, that the woman who gave me the bottle of Beaujolais looks at me smiling, and says:

- "I gave you the bottle because I love you."
- "Nothing more to say, *chérie*" – I answer, picking the bottle up from the small coffee table and amidst the silence of all those figures in the room, she and I take our leave. As we do, we see a gold-tinged vineyard flowing down the hillside as the resplendent sun sets in Burgundy.

Fourth criterion: a discourse is a coherent system of meanings

Analytical step number 7: identify the different versions or images of the social worlds that co-exist in the text

We can ponder at least five rather covert, or implicit, *social worlds* interwoven into my bottle of Beaujolais; worlds autonomous yet somehow complementary, perhaps linked by the very liquidity of the wine; activated, capriciously, as my palate savours sips of this red libation and/or as some of the realities enveloped in the product come into consciousness.

The first to emerge in my mind is the *social world of tradition, both family and Burgundy entrepreneurship*, with its production of wines of consistently high quality; a world that embraces care and love for the homeland; a proud lineage; past and future concentrated in wine and its ecological condition, including, as well, Burgundy's climate, the casks where the wine ages, the internationalization of the product and the economic prosperity generated by the efforts, talents and diligence of fieldworkers, oenologists and managers.

Also tangible is the *social world of patronage of local culture, the pulse of economic development and the benefits that accrue to community and region*: the company's elegant generosity expressed through sensitivity proffered and the promotion of deeply-rooted cultural values; sponsoring and promoting a literary award to exalt the grape, the wine and a certain *lifestyle*; support for Burgundy's literary club; philanthropy; financing the yearly classical music festival and the singers who participate; backing the international festival for *suspense* cinema in Beaune; hospitality, cultural dinners amidst books, canapés and cocktails.

Close on the heels of that world, I perceive the *social world of pleasure and maturity of living*: good food; glamour and discrete, subtly aristocratic, elegance; the love of nature idealized by a friendly community in a kind of bubble of harmony that surrounds bitterness and the problems of the world; aromas of intense fruit and pleasures of voluptuousness; floral notes of existence; wine coupled with meat, cheese and sweetbread; the lovely smile of that unknown young woman; quails stuffed with *dauphinoise* potatoes; gardens illuminated by night; and apples, plums; the city discovered; the memories.

Tenuously, yet with sufficient clarity, looms the *social world of responsibility in caring for the health of those who consume the wine*: the warnings about alcohol content and possible "severe consequences" for the "health of children" or of pregnant women who consume the rich liquid.

Finally, from the translucent heart of this bottle of Beaujolais arises – how could it not – dressed in characteristic red tones, the *social world of the promise of happiness and erotic love*: imaginings of the wonder of naked bodies under white sheets, near wooden window frames, a swatch of sky and sun we breathe; the mystery of travel; the silent gaze; the far-off landscape; sweet anxiety; the piano one hears, the kisses that do not return.

Analytical step number 8: identify the implicit cultural rules that articulate the worlds appearing in the text and then speculate on how to best confront the text's own discourses or attend to possible objections to its terminology

What a situation! This is getting complicated! Another sip of wine. Cheers. All right ... now I can state that one of the first implicit cultural rules holds that (in principle) industrial wine production – especially French – must be upheld, for its own benefit, for its worldwide importance, especially when this production salvages geographic-ecological traditions of such high quality as the case of Burgundy wines. I mean, industrial wine production generates jobs and economic *prosperity* and consolidates social tissues (at least in France). Anyone who opposes this criterion is (at least) irresponsible, an ignoramus, a subject devoid of all economic-entrepreneurial sensitivity. Because, really, can we impugn the global success of such productive projects? Do companies like this one really destroy the planet? Who could blame *Monsieur* Alberic Bichot, the current General Director of this wine-making house, for the awful ills that afflict the world?

A second implicit rule in this context is that all successful enterprises must be "socially responsible" and "culturally sensitive" to their historical-geographic milieu; must promote collective development and stimulate and support diverse artistic and cultural expressions. And, if it's about producing red wine, they must also love and promote literature, music and cinema, for who consumes wine more devotedly than poets, bohemians, and intellectuals? It's really hard to beautify the world while drinking vulgar beer. And water, that's only for survival. Banish the thought of mentioning the ignominy of contaminating one's blood and soul-consuming *Coca-Cola* and junk food while flooding the brain with network TV rubbish, as so sadly occurs in my troubled country.

Another area of cultural meaning implicit in the bottle of Beaujolais (one often besieged by certain institutions devoted to maintaining health and the social order) is the capacity to experience renewed pleasure in living or, better, the ability to continually renew oneself; a delicate ability fostered, precisely, by consuming red wine and, clearly, by the bottle of wine I find myself enjoying at this moment, especially when it comes to my hands as the gift of an alluring woman. Renewing oneself demands somehow exchanging the bitterness of death for the vigour of living. And here wine, can surely help out because, as Roland Barthes writes:

(wine) is, above all, a substance of conversion, capable of altering situations and states, and extracting from objects their opposite, making, for instance, the weak strong, the reticent chatterboxes; this is the origin of its ancient alquimic legacy, its philosophical power to transmute, or create, *ex nihilo*.[10]

Thus, this bottle of Beaujolais opens us up to desire, play, laughter, eroticism, the very intensity of life, so those who might impugn this truth of existence, can be none other than those strange, grey beings, marked undoubtedly by sadness; those we know as *abstainers*.

Of course, there is another implicit cultural rule; this one stipulating – through warning labels – that people who consume wine must care for their health. The goal is to prevent alcoholism, congenital malformations and traffic accidents. Officials of health institutions and individuals who champion virtue and benevolence heartily applaud these instructions.

The other prescriptive sense perceptible in the bottle of Beaujolais emerges as one appreciates the interconnection of things and situations, for the bottle itself is designed to somehow generate, invent, promote, or facilitate the sublime moment of erotic love, that love which opens like a spring flower. Who could receive the gift of a bottle of Beaujolais without thinking at that instant of the possibility of having sex with someone (or something)? Now, people who have no wish to provoke such thoughts in others shouldn't be giving out bottles of Beaujolais; it seems to me they'd be better off, giving, perhaps, a self-help book, a chronometer, an ashtray, a *monkey wrench*, or a tyre.[11] Objections to this other milieu of the production of subjectivity present in the bottle of Beaujolais can only have their origin in the desolation of anorgasmia.

Fifth criterion: one discourse refers to other discourses

Analytical steps numbers 9 and 10: identify the contrasts between the distinct forms of speech and the occasions in which they overlap or are superimposed

As pointed out in *Analytical step number 4* of this reflection, in the bottle of Beaujolais there co-exist different styles and forms of speech, or discourse, that through their complexity generate a very important network of cultural and symbolic identity, but that also contrast due to their intrinsic meaning such that they may overlap or be superimposed upon others to reveal their contradictions or the thematic and political distance between them. As an example we have that noble, distinguished form or style of speaking typical of traditional French elegance (a certain discrete opulence and subtly arrogant gesture), the gold lettering, the aristocratic pride, the coat-of-arms, have nothing to do with the – *so* ordinary and plebian – *biopolitically*-motivated technical-scientific expressions that appear on the bottle due to legal obligations, manifested in the excessively-discrete, almost occult, mode in which they are placed on a microscopic fringe of the main label. Then we have the form or style of professional speech plus that of product quality control, which seem to adjectivize the substantive aristocratic meaning of the elegant, opulent and traditional discursive form of this French wine-making house, materialized and symbolized in the bottle of Beaujolais.

Sixth criterion: a discourse is reflected in its own way of speaking

Analytical step number 11: make comparisons with other texts and evaluate how these forms of speech are directed to distinct audiences

Although it is useful to analyse the discourses of other bottles of Beaujolais, at this moment and with the creative lucidity created by the formidable wine I am enjoying, I can state that the patterns of meaning displayed in the discourses of this particular bottle operate in many symbolic spaces and levels, articulating the specific values and practices of distinct publics. The various social sectors that participate in consuming and/or commercializing such products can discern messages that seem appropriate, stimulating, or pleasing to their particular modes of conceiving the world, their priorities, and their criteria for the possibility of – and right to – obtain, imbibe, or offer the wine contained in the bottle. Much could be clarified in this regard by the work of designing the labels, the product's presentation, and the marketing lines and publicity campaigns suggested by the bottle of Beaujolais.

Perhaps the seigneurial, aristocratic style that predominates in the presentation reflects the crisis that the "new Beaujolais" (to which I shall return below) experienced due to its lower quality, excessive production and low consumption compared to previous years, and that generated the association of wine from this region with a cheap, intranscendent product. In reaction, winemakers chose to redesign their processes and bet on wines of higher quality, class and depth but without sacrificing the *joyous nature* that impregnates the Beaujolais region. Thus, "facing the reduced consumption of the *new Beaujolais*, winemakers put their money on serious wines of cheerful nature".[12] Whatever the case, the traditional, aristocratic, distinguished style of discourse on the bottle connects, perfectly and positively, with certain intellectual sectors of Latin America's middle classes (whose cultural and recreational pretensions are far beyond the reach of their real economic possibilities – as in my case, I'm afraid), with young Japanese executives desirous of going out for fun with their – female – friends on a formal-gown night in Tokyo, with Californian musicians out to participate in a gay nostalgia party in San Francisco, or with Swiss heads-of-household organizing an elegant picnic with their kids.

The professional style and quality control proudly reflected in other messages on the bottle can easily seduce North American, French, or Chinese distributors who seek to acquire the product to do business through distribution and sales.

And, finally, the technical scientific form or style of the discourse manifested in the more discrete messages on the bottle of Beaujolais seems to be addressed to all those English, German, or Danish scrutinizers, activists of healthy practices and vigilantes of virtue who carefully peruse the product's technical and sanitary data before deciding whether or not to drink or recommend it.

Analytical step number 12: reflect upon and select the adequate terminology for naming or describing the discourses articulated in the text

Based on the reflection posited in analytical steps 4 and 7 of this analysis, and in an attempt to summarize what has been said, we can identify three broad discursive lines on the bottle of Beaujolais that we might call, in order of importance:

1. The traditional, aristocratic discourse of this wine-making family of Burgundy;
2. The professional discourse of wine quality; and
3. The technical-sanitary discourse of modern-day wine production.

Discussion

Discourse analysis can be conceived as a variant of the kind of qualitative research that demands recovering its reflexive aspects. As Ian Parker points out, one must clarify that the reading offered is nothing more than my reaction to the text (in this case the text-bottle of Beaujolais) and that discourses are both products of our creation and "objects" that exist independently of us. The encounter with these discourses, as this text manifests, is not an encounter with something unknown, but quite the contrary. The history that defines discourses and that sustains them as "objective" phenomena is also the history that defines us as "subjective" beings (...). Our subjectivity as historical product and contingent form is, therefore, a research instrument of maximum value for decodifying language.[13]

In any case, I must add that at this juncture of the analysis, I am writing under the cheering effects of this formidable "juice of sun and earth" as Gastón Bachelard might say.[14] While drinking the wine I make an ostentation of pleasure, though my intention, or objective, is not to become inebriated because, as Roland Barthes has observed, in France (and this goes for my home as well), "drunkenness is a consequence, *never* the finality" (...) "wine is not only a filter, it is also the ongoing act of drinking, the *gesture* has a decorative value and the power of the wine can never be separated from its modes of existence" (...).[15]

Seventh criterion: a discourse is historically-localized

Analytical step number 13: study where, how and when the discourses in the text emerge

Spurred by the urge to advance in the elaboration of this analysis, I can see clearly that the discourses of the bottle of Beaujolais emerge in the French entrepreneurial settings of wine-making in the heat of the historical need to strengthen the commercial placement of the product worldwide and to modify its image to reflect greater seriousness and higher category. *Beaujolais* thus became both a cultural phenomenon and a business of great importance. The denomination of origin "Beaujolais", by the way, was officially recognized by French authorities in 1937, but Parisians did not begin to consume it in large quantities until the 1950s, the British in the 1960s, and Americans in the 1980s, the period that marked, especially for the *nouveau Beaujolais*, the high-point of its popularity in world commerce, propelled by important creative *marketing* processes that made "*Le Beaujolais nouveau est arrivé!*" the expression that year-after-year, in the third week of November, announced France's collective festival to present and distribute this young wine to the country and the whole world, according to the tradition begun, precisely, in the 1950s. In fact, a novel by René Fallet published in 1975 bears this title, as does a film that premiered in 1978.

Once these conditions had been created, those years transformed the *nouveau Beaujolais* into a highly-coveted product whose consumption in developed countries shot demand up to unprecedented levels that surpassed available supplies. Seeking to take advantage of this "fever for *nouveau*", many Beaujolais producers began to churn out huge amounts of this young, fruity, light-to-the-palate wine (a light liquid, lacking transcendence, of smooth *bouquet* and an aftertaste sweetened with hints of gooseberry and raspberry, so attractive to undemanding consumers), though this decreased production of the traditional, high-quality Beaujolais with its better structure and seriousness (like the one I sip as I write). It has been noted that around 1988, for example, 60% of the basic denomination of Beaujolais corresponded to the *nouveau* type: "Winemakers gathered the grapes early, when only minimally mature, adding sugar to the juice to raise the alcohol content; thus maximizing yields".[16]

The problem emerged when, a few years later – in the late 1990s and early 2000s – a reaction against the *nouveau Beaujolais* began to emerge among consumers because, apparently, at that moment the whole *Beaujolais* brand had developed a poor reputation: "The *nouveau* has destroyed our image (...) all Beaujolais is now confounded with the *nouveau* (...) the *nouveau* really contributed to the problems here", certain producers exclaimed.[17] According to some data, after the 2001 harvest, a surplus of over a million boxes of low-quality wine had accumulated; impossible to sell because the market was flooded. Producers found themselves forced to either distil or destroy their stocks.[18]

The response of wineries was to rethink their production strategies for Beaujolais; in effect opting to produce more complex wines that required longer "aging" in oaken casks before being bottled and consumed. The goal was to make "serious wines of cheerful nature"; that is, wines from a region by then well-known for offering light, jovial, smooth liquids, but that now set out to produce wines characterized by depth and class (*serious wines*) conceived to recover the category, lineage, tradition and consistently-high quality in French and international contexts. To achieve this, wine-makers encouraged the production of regional, or homeland, wines (*terruño* in Spanish, *terroir* in French) in special vineyards, seeking to achieve sustainable wine-making operations that respected "natural equilibriums", and used only ploughs and organic fertilization. The whole process had to be as unobtrusive as possible, using oaken casks to achieve a finished product that would be an expressive, authentic wine of elegant character.

Such an expansive re-orientation of wineries in Beaujolais surely demanded modifying how they would be articulated discursively, so the work of re-designing the presentation, texts and images on the label, as well as *marketing* strategies had to be elaborated from different coordinates and generate distinct existential plexuses in order to conquer more stable markets. To position the product and achieve good sales, it would no longer suffice (and, it appears, would not be *convenient*) to appeal only to the frivolity of social fiestas, happy faces and multi-coloured balloons. No, this required opening other worlds, other complexities and desires, evocations and aspirations that would permit sensing the wine as a river of subjective profundities that reaffirm life's beauty and enthusiasm, love reborn, and the possibility of sharing our time on Earth with dignity and elegance. Of course, I don't know how many – or just what – inter-subjective effects the discourses articulated on the bottle of Beaujolais we're analysing may have achieved, but I would emphasize the recovery of their inevitably *aristocratic* character and the concomitance with certain vitalistic attitudes that are revealed and potentiated upon drinking the wine it contains.

Analytical step number 14: describe how the discourses present in the text operate by "naturalizing" their referents

Of course, everything written on the bottle of Beaujolais is naturalized in the sense that no one questions its presumed intrinsic value, the legitimacy of its positionings and messages, the importance – even necessity – of phrasing them in just that way and at that precise moment. In reality, in many everyday life situations, everyone – all of us – naturalize what we say. *Analyzing* something is, in and of itself, an important way of de-naturalizing that reality (I can't imagine how terrible it would be to go around *de-naturalizing* everything we say at every moment, though I can swear that in certain particularly obstinate intellectual and analytical sectors, everything is naturalized eventually, even the exercise of striving, at all costs, to "de-naturalize" everything that is thought). This is why one more naturalization shouldn't be criticized too harshly.

But added to the foregoing, it occurs that somehow (at least for me at this moment), what the bottle of Beaujolais says will indeed have intrinsic value, legitimacy and pertinence. After all, is it not simply natural that a magnificent red wine like the one I am sipping, produced by the prestigious *House of Albert Bichot* (that has always been there), should place the gold family coat-of-arms on its label with unleashed dogs guarding the forest and the deer under the nine-pointed crown? And, of course, is it not also natural that those who produce the wine do so in a most professional, serious manner, to safeguard the health of us all? Could anyone dare to doubt this? Let's see, it's not only that this is natural, it is in fact *necessary* that this wine be so formidable. Every time that a sip passes through my throat, I travel to the south of Burgundy, walk its endearing landscapes that rejuvenate my body, while something like a superior lineage, a sidereal excitement, courses through my veins. What I mean to say is that drinking this wine transforms you, naturally, into a *prince*.

Eighth criterion: discourses sustain and/or subvert institutions

Analytical step number 15: examine how implicit discourses reproduce and reinforce this or that institution

One can appreciate, through the description presented herein, that the implicit discourses on the bottle of Beaujolais reproduce and reinforce various institutions: above all, fortifying and vindicating *the French and Burgundian entrepreneurial wine-making institution*; consolidated as well in *the cultural institution of the aristocratic values linked to distinction and good taste in the traditional consumption of red wine*; while also strengthening *the institution of professionalism and quality control in the elaboration of the product*. We might add that, though perhaps only indirectly, the discourses and social worlds implied in the bottle of Beaujolais sustain and project other cultural institutions, like those involving *publicity, marketing and graphic design in the wine industry and trade*. Also, subtly but with great import, this vindicates the institution (or *myth*, as Barthes would say) of *social co-existence and integration, together with the pleasure and maturity of living, all articulated by the shared consumption of red wine*. Barthes explains this perfectly:

> Believing in wine is an act of collective compulsion: the Frenchman who would distance himself from the myth finds himself experiencing problems of integration, not severe, but clear; the first would consist, precisely, in the need to give explanations (...) [for] society classifies those who do not believe in wine as ill, defective or

impaired: it does not *understand* them (...). In contrast, those who perform the practice of [sipping] wine obtain a diploma for good integration: *knowing how* to drink is a national technique that functions to rate the French, demonstrating simultaneously their power of actuation, their control and their sociability. In this way, wine establishes a moral collective in whose interior all things are recouped: excesses, misfortunes, crimes, are, without doubt, possible with wine, but never, no way, evil, perfidy or ugliness; the evil it can engender enters into that of fatality and escape and, therefore, punishment; it constitutes an evil of theater, not an evil of temperament.[19]

Finally, it vindicates – how could it not – the cultural and psycho-social institution of *the engendering and fantasy of love and sexuality sustained and propelled by the gift and the shared consumption of the wine*, as long as, of course, the process takes place when one dreams or is in the presence of someone (or any type of *post-person*) that one likes, probably someone young and beautiful; or in the presence of someone for whom one may feel attraction of an erotic nature that, by its very condition and beyond its springlike temple, seems in-explicable.[20] Whatever the case, it brings to mind these verses from Louis Aragon:

> And the night awoke as a warm young woman (...)
> Shall we not recover life oh false deceased,
> for it is a door that opens at last because it is
> spring that arrives at last with its perfume
> that touches the wind like a caress
> For whom, however, the flowers but for you whom I loved
> With the most beautiful spring I would not know what to do
> Without you the most beautiful April the sweetest May
> Without you they are nothing more than grief, without you they
> are nothing more than Hell (...).[21]

Or, more directly, this suggestion from André Frénaud:

> The craziest one will possess my life
> We shall drink it while singing
> in the rivers in the afternoon air (...).[22]

Analytical step number 16: explore how the discourses present in the text attack or subvert one institution or another

Implicitly, the discourses that appear on the bottle of Beaujolais and the social worlds configured through them subvert, or impugn, in my view, at least three lines of discursive-institutional prescription currently in vogue, and often articulated and infiltrated (in different ways and with unequal impact), in the subjectivity of any one of us:

Above all, they oppose *the institutional practice – biopolitical in nature – of seeing abstinence from alcohol as a sign of sanity, for this promotes a condition of sobriety while also preventing accidents and diverse diseases (that entail costs for public health systems when they occur), as well as conflicts and the physical, psychological and social damage that alcoholism produces.* In fact, recent years have witnessed the consolidation of an institutional process designed to dissuade people from drinking wine, even in France,

> To the extent that government officials often group wine with other alcoholic drinks as a threat to public health, the aggressive measures deployed in France to combat drinking while under the influence now mean that even a couple glasses of wine with dinner will put the individual over the legal limit. Moreover, a neo-prohibitionist attitude has risen above the most common discourse regarding wine. Today, France is discussing the issue of raising taxes on wine and restricting conversations and publicity involving this product in the social media and Internet. Health officials say the objective is to combat growing rates of alcoholism. Those in the wine business [however] believe that alcoholism is due to the increased consumption of liquor and binge-drinking. Americans have learned much from the French about the pleasures of living. Today, [the French] are learning from the United States how to control [those very pleasures].[23]

The bottle of Beaujolais, with its implicit discourses and social worlds, also – somehow – challenges *the ethical-political practice instituted by some anti-capitalist groups, of fomenting austerity and militant asceticism in favour of some collective libertarian cause or another,* because for these "revolutionaries" it is always the case – depending on the context in which they operate – that drinking a good French wine is rather a shameful and intolerable thing to do because its production entails, unfortunately, consolidating capitalist wine-making companies and, hence, the spurious enrichment of a handful of men astute in building businesses who care not a hoot for the poor and downtrodden peoples of the planet; peoples who for a myriad of historical, economic and social reasons, could hardly – or likely wouldn't even want – to drink, for pleasure only, the wine of which we are speaking; peoples upon whom capitalist expansion imposes very different ways of being and of consuming to the detriment of their traditions (though wine itself is in no way to blame). Here, once again, allow me to paraphrase Emma Goldman: "if I can't *drink a bottle of Beaujolais*, then it ain't my revolution". Whatever the case, Barthes words will elucidate the issue:

> For it is true that wine is a substance both beautiful and good, but no less true that its production participates squarely in French capitalism, whether that of the warehousers or of the grand Algerian colonists who impose upon the Muslims, who have no bread to eat, a strange culture on the same lands of which he has just been dispossessed (...). So the characteristic of our current alienation is that wine, precisely, cannot be a completely happy substance, except when one, unduly, forgets that it is, as well, a product of expropriation.[24]

Without doubt, the discourses and social worlds enveloped in the bottle of Beaujolais in some way subvert *that – fortunately, not overly successful – cultural institution of moral puritanism (of Jewish-Christian and Calvinist origins) and its alliances with virtue and sexual modesty that favour an exacerbated spirituality linked to practices of chastity and the renouncement of all earthly pleasures.* Here, I refer to that series of prescriptions, values and customs, more-or-less subterranean and extended, micro-physical in nature, that frame life in terms of penitence, abstinence and all manner of mortifications of the flesh, for they assume (often quite hypocritically) "human nature" to be a corrupt, depraved condition. The result is this yearning to be rigorously virtuous, even puritanical, and vehemently oppose the temptations of concupiscence to the point that good conscience deems necessary. One should not smoke, nor eat to excess, nor drink wine to laugh and feel content. Perhaps the only acceptable way for such champions of temperance, prudence and humility to actually partake of

this libation is understanding it as the symbol of the blood of Christ in the context of ritual practice, since ingesting it under all other circumstance promotes drunkenness, the vice that will befall one (according to the *Dictionary of Values, Virtues and Vices* that I consulted) as a consequence of intentionally excessive consumption of wine despite one's clear awareness of the drink's possible effects. "In this case – so people say – drunkenness is a cardinal sin of the genre 'gluttony', a category that distinguishes feasts from boozing and inebriation" (...).[25] But, I ask myself, what might all those good-thinking individuals say of the explicit, precious sensuality that is so closely-associated with wine, as revealed in the very *Song of Songs*, whence we extract, to complete the point, a few fragments:
She:

> That he may kiss me with kisses from his mouth!
> Your love is an exquisite wine,
> Smooth is the aroma of your perfumes
> Your name, a balsam that spills over (...).
> We remember your caresses, better than wine
> No wonder you are so loved! (...).
> He took me to a wine cellar
> And placed upon me his insignia, which was love
> Pass me some raisin cake
> Re-animate me with apples
> for I am afflicted by love (...).

He:

> How loving are your caresses
> My sister, my love,
> How Delicious your love!
> Yes, so much better than wine!
> And the aroma of your perfumes
> Cannot be compared with any other.
> The lips of my love distill pure honey;
> Under your tongue
> Are found milk and honey
> And the fragrance of your garments
> Is that of the forests of Lebanon (...).
> I have entered my orchard

My sister, my love,
I have taken my myrrh with my perfume,
I have eaten my honey from its honeycomb
I have drunk my wine and my milk.
Friends, eat, drink,
Oh my dear ones! Drink til you are drunk (...).
May your breasts be as clusters of grapes
And your breath as the perfume of apples!
May your words be as generous as wine,
That go straight to your love
Flowing from your lips as you sleep (...).[26]

Ninth criterion: discourses reproduce power relations

Analytical steps number 17 and 18: examine which people gain or benefit from the discourses present in the text and so desire to support and promote them; and which lose something, or could be harmed by those discourses, and so wish to discredit or dissolve them

A simple question: who profits, or benefits, in one way or another, from and/or would seek to support and promote these discourses? Well, the owners of the family business; producers and work teams; publicists; merchants; oenologists; intellectuals seeking contentment; those – men or women – who have sex with a beautiful woman (or simply have sex); the literati; lovers; composers of verse or music, or those who paint pictures; friends of both sexes who get together to laugh; restauranteurs and folk who promote Mediterranean gastronomy; romantics of both sexes; people who enjoy good health; those who know how to have fun; or those that – in the words of the bard – "make worlds and dreams".[27]

On the other hand, there are those who feel in some way harmed and/or wish to discredit or dissolve these discourses: abstainers; puritans; militant ascetics; people who suffer from anorgasmia; those who cannot drink wine because they are ill; technocrats in the health sector; soft drink industrialists; authoritarians; despots; police that must control the frenzy of a party; anti-alcoholism scientificists, and/or those subjects who know not refinement and delicacy.

Tenth criterion: discourses have ideological effects

Analytical steps 19 and 20: to show how these implicit discourses are linked to other discourses that sustain and vindicate power relations (or how they articulate with the possibility of resisting power), and how they reproduce or subvert dominant conceptions and the possibilities of change they provide

In these final steps, I offer a rather more relaxed and free reflection because, as the reader may have noticed, at this point I don't believe I can demonstrate anything with my arguments; though perhaps I can intone, with the ancient poets, "the elegant song of Mr. Baco, struck as my mind is by the rays of the wine".[28]

In its heterogeneous discursive articulation and the networks of meaning it promotes, the bottle of Beaujolais somehow responds to a kind of urgency to live and is etched into the interplay of power relations and resistance to power, such that, as a result, it is linked to diverse productions and relations of knowledge. It generates a certain *positivity* understood as a socio-material nucleus that implies values, rules, rituals, and institutions that, in turn, involve different sentiments, affections, beliefs and individual opinions; that is, in its discourses and associated social worlds, the bottle of Beaujolais presupposes and displays processes of subjectification, of de-subjectification and of the production of complex, diverse and intense subjectivities. Thus, I myself as subject analyst (*Latin-euro-cosmopoli-urban*[29] analyst) am something produced and eventually negated by the bottle while, from my person, there hatches, simultaneously, a *multiverse* of subjective contradictory possibilities, a Baroque imaginary, and a potency of invention of worlds. Through the bottle of Beaujolais one can somehow create, govern or control existence; though this can also be oriented and re-oriented, and anyone's emotions, behaviours, gestures and ideas can be re-constituted or re-created.

Nor is the bottle of Beaujolais a coincidence or accident of culture; no, it is the result of a multivocal process of unpredictable humanization of the world that might presuppose and involve in its birth and development, in its emergence and projection, a desire for joy; a propensity towards jubilation; a possible (or virtual) happiness captured in the very materiality of the object and its discourses.

Is in this context that, through Giorgio Agamben's reflection, I can come to understand what is constituted as the first, and perhaps most important, closure of the present study: *the bottle of Beaujolais is a dispositive* (*Yahoo*! Wow, now I'm really plastered! Allow me to send affectionate greetings to my friends – male and female – of the *Ambulant, Transdisciplinary Seminar on Critical Thought and Fictions* in Morelia and the folks at my favourite tavern, *El Barrio*). But, we must carry on, for Agamben writes:

> I shall use the term 'dispositive' for, literally, any thing that somehow has the ability to capture, orient, determine, intercept, model, control and ensure the gestures, behaviors, opinions and discourses of living beings. Therefore, not only prisons, madhouses, the Panoptic, schools, confession, factories, disciplines, juridical measures, etc., whose connection with power is somehow evident, but also the pen, writing, literature, philosophy, agriculture, the cigarette, navigation, computers, mobile phones and – why not? – language itself, which may be the most ancient of all dispositives, in which thousands and thousands of years ago a primate – probably never realizing the consequences of its actions – was so unaware that he allowed himself to be trapped.[30]

And I, as a living being, have been entrapped by the bottle of Beaujolais, a dispositive. In my defence, I could say that this is a dispositive which allows me to savour a very good wine. But, the analysis does not end here. For as we know, Agamben proposes dividing all things that exist into two broad groups: *living beings* (or *substances*) on the one hand, and *dispositives*, on the other. And it is from the relations between the living and dispositives that *subjects* emerge. The living and subjects are super-imposed, but not totally:

> In this sense, for example, one specific individual, one specific substance, can be the site of multiple processes of subjectification: the mobile telephone user, the Internet surfer, the short story writer, those who are passionate about the tango, the *non-global*, etc. To the enormous growth of dispositives in our time there corresponds a similarly enormous proliferation of processes of subjectification.[31]

Nonetheless, according to Agamben, this situation does not mean the loss or annulment of subjectivity as a category and as potential for transformation but, rather, an unpredictable multiplication and dissemination of it. In fact, in the face of the huge accumulation and proliferation of dispositives and their ubiquitous presence and action in the lives of individuals, the question that arises is how to confront them and the meaning that the answer might have for intimate, collective existence. Following this logic, Agamben proposes that the strategy for confronting dispositives must consist in freeing *that which has been trapped* to return it or *restitute it for a possible common use*. To this end, he adopts the term *pro-fanation*.[32] In effect, Roman juridical and religious culture assumed that sacred or religious things are those that – in one way or another – pertain to the gods and, due to this condition, are impeded from forming part of the free use and commerce in the world of the human. The act of *con-secrating* refers, precisely, to the moment at which something leaves the world of the human to enter the world of the gods, and this step – this separation – always entails sacrifice. *Sacrilege*, in contrast, is the trans-gression of the condition of the sacred. And *profanation*, finally, is the act by virtue of which something is returned or restored from the celestial or sacred sphere to the use and property of human beings; that is to say, profanation "is the *counter-dispositive* that restores to common use that which sacrifice had once separated and divided".[33]

Well then, this brings us to the second conclusion of our analysis: **the bottle of Beaujolais is something sacred**. It was produced through a ritual of sacrifice and separation from the human; that is, a ritual process through which that object found itself suddenly extracted from the common use of mortals and transferred to the sphere of the divine, to the world of dreams and of hopes: in effect, when you look at the bottle of Beaujolais and hold it in your hands, you touch, literally, the materiality of the gods and can feel for an instant its oh so distant, but incredibly intense, promise.

But if, as Agamben says, "that which has been ritually separated, can be restored through ritual to the profane sphere"[34] then no doubt exists, and what emerges – when all is said and done – is the third conclusion: **the bottle of Beaujolais must be profaned by the act of drinking it**. And with that, this contact, this exultation, this interplay, we succeed in having the gods contained in its interior pass into the blood that courses through our human veins, and so can usher in that endearing, libertarian and plethoric world of inventions and potencies called *enthusiasm*.

Limits and Critiques

The analysis of the discourse presented herein suffers from the most serious of all possible problems: discovering that, at the end of the process, no actual analysis of the discourse was made (at least none that is plausible or that contributes anything new), but perhaps only a *divertissement*, an irresponsible play of meanings, an invention made of words, or simply a bunch of gibberish. The harshest criticism, surely, would be one that points out the text's unscrupulously delirious, vitalist, recreational, fanciful, and speculative character, of the kind that is so profoundly useless for any scientific, political or social cause. Added to this, the text – while pretending to entertain – is filled with seriousness throughout its development; for this reason it turns out to be, as well, highly incongruent. Without doubt, the good consciences of some moralism – or other – could react to the text with various forms of hostility; for example: claiming that it promotes consuming alcohol; or that it offends all of Christianity's fine sensibilities; or that it reaffirms or enthrones the *heterosexual matrix* (obvious, since the analyst boasts of having a girlfriend or wife with whom he is quite happily traversing the south of France); or that it is an apologia (and then mockery) of France's entrepreneurial wine-making world; or that it is disrespectful of the sincere efforts of discourse analysis in academic and political scenarios (especially Ian Parker, who bears not the slightest bit of blame for what has been done in this text); or that deep down it speaks superficially, nay frivolously, from a certain solipsism and self-referentiality and that, definitively, the author, aside from being an intranscendent individual, has a particularly nasty propensity towards imagination and dipsomania.

Epilogue

The woman who gave me the bottle of Beaujolais and I made love in an enchanting villa on the coast, quite near Montpellier, the afternoon descending with its golden lights. The empty bottle sitting upon an elevated terrace, facing the sea.

> The empty bottle should speak with the waves. It is a locus of rumor that should be echoed in the agitated sea. She is –audacious paradox – in charge of verticality in the face of the undulations of the maritime horizon. Promoted to the rank of the center of the universe, she has the dignity, majesty, of a cosmic verticality (...). That empty bottle is a globe of fire, the clouds in the sky nothing more than the gloom of its shadow. The cosmic bottle, the brilliant bottle, has obtained vision, it sees far (...). All things are raised to the heights through the grace of limits (...). In the solitude facing the sea, the bottle exasperates its height; calls to the zenith, to the rocks, to the forest. And the buttresses, councilors of terrestrial prudence, well they are pulled towards the sky. They shall remain standing through the stream of their crazy imprudence.[35]

Notes

1 I have developed some of these ideas in: García, R. (2008) *El diálogo en descomposición*. Mexico: AMAPSI/ UMSNH, pp. 55–63.

2 Parker, I. (1992) *Discourse Dynamics: Critical Analysis for Social and Individual Psychology*. London: Routledge.

3 Parker, I. *Op. cit.* pp. 6–7. On this topic, see also the magnificent article: Pavón-Cuéllar, D. (2011) La psicología crítica de Ian Parker: análisis del discurso, marxismo trotskista y psicoanálisis lacaniano. In: *Teoría y crítica de la psicología* 1, 56–82. Available at www.teocripsi.com

4 See: Parker, I. (1996) Discurso, cultura y poder en la vida cotidiana. In: Gordo, A.; Linaza, J. (Comps.) (1996) *Psicologías, discurso y poder (PDP)*. Madrid: Visor, pp. 79–92.

5 Estatuto de la Viña del Vino y los Alcoholes, article 10 (cited in: Pastor, A. (1990) *Diccionario del vino y la cava*. Barcelona: Fomento comercio editorial S. L./ Editorial Hermes, p. 301).

6 In his works on *Actor Network Theory* (ANT), Mike Michael proposes the concept of "ethno-epistemic assemblages". See, for example: Ethno-Epistemic Assemblages: Heterogeneity and Relationality in Scientific Citizenship. In: Irwin, A.; Michael, M. (Eds.) (2003) *Science, Social Theory and Public Knowledge*. Open University Press.

7 Huidobro, V. (1919) Fragment of the poem "Canto II". In: *Altazor*. Madrid: Compañía Ibero Americana de Publicaciones, S.A., 1931, p. 17.

8 Borges, J. L. (1977) Fragments of the poem "Las causas". In: *Historia de la noche*. From *Jorge Luis Borges. Poesía y prosa*. Mexico: Promexa, pp. 237–238.

9 "In Burgundy, a vineyard is always surrounded by a wall called a *clos*". See: "El clos de Vougeot: el microcosmos católico de Borgoña" In: Dominé, A. (2004) *El vino*. Barcelona: Könemann, pp. 185, 193.

10 Barthes, R. (1957, 1980) *Mitologías*. Mexico: Siglo XXI, 2008, p. 75.

11 Although these two latter objects (the monkey wrench and automobile tyre), may also come to be related with pronounced lubricious or amorous thoughts, as can be seen in the magnificent Brazilian porn movie entitled *Mechanic getting involved in threesome*. Available at: www.xvideos.com

12 See: www.mercadosdelvino.com *El Beaujolais planea nuevos rumbos* 1/12/2007. Accessed 4/01/2016.

13 Parker, I. (1996) Discurso, cultura y poder en la vida cotidiana. In: Gordo, A.; Linaza, J. (Comps.) (1996) *Psicologías, discurso y poder (PDP)*. Madrid: Visor, p.87.

14 Bachelard, G. cited by Barthes, R. *Op. cit.* p. 75.

15 Barthes, R. *Op. cit.* p. 76.

16 See: *El Beaujolais planea nuevos rumbos*. In: www.mercadosdelvino.com 1/12/ 2007. Accessed 4/01/2016.

17 *Idem.*

18 See: ¿Le Beaujolais nouveau est passé? In: https://chezlafayette.worldpress.com. Accessed 24/11/2014.

19 Barthes, R. *Op. cit.* pp. 76–77.

20 In this regard, we can review an interesting note entitled: "El consumo moderado de vino tinto mejora el deseo sexual de las mujeres", at: www. elmundo.es 3/12/2009. Accessed 15/09/2016. The note is based on a study by the Universities of Torino and Florence (published – it says – in the *Journal of Sexual Medicine*). It concludes, among other things, that "women who drink

one or two cups of wine daily obtain better scores for sexual desire, lubrication, and the sexual function in general". With such scientific support, no doubt can exist as to the importance of offering a cup of wine, or two, at the hour of seduction.

21 Aragon, L. Fragment of the poem "La primavera". In: Díaz, S. (Selec.) (1985) *Poesía de amor francesa.* Havana: Editorial Arte y Literatura, pp. 209–211.

22 Frénaud, A. Fragment of the poem "La más loca". In: Díaz, S. *Op. cit.* p. 135.

23 See: Los europeos se apartan del consumo de vinos. In: www.nacion.com 12/12/2013. Accessed 10/08/2016.

24 Barthes, R. *Op. cit.* p. 78.

25 García, L.; Saíz, M. (2007) *Diccionario de valores, virtudes y vicios.* Mexico: Trillas, p. 75.

26 *Cantar de los cantares.* La Biblia. Latinoamérica. Madrid: Ediciones Paulinas. Verbo divino, 1972, pp. 884–893.

27 Fernández Retamar, R. (1970) Fragment of the poem: "Felices los normales". In: *A quien pueda interesar (Poesía, 1958–1970).* Mexico: Siglo XXI, p. 64.

28 Verses by Arquíloco. The complete fragment prays: *Bacchi Regis canticum elegans Dityrambicum auspicari scio, Vini fulmina percussa mente* ("I know how to begin the dithyramb, the elegant song of Lord Bacchus, as my mind is struck by the rays of the wine"). Cited in Ripa, Cesare (1593, 1987, 2002) *Iconología.* Madrid: Akal, Vol. II, p. 346.

29 The term is from Juan Gelman, who uses it in the poem "Conversaciones". See: Gelman, J. (1968) *Poemas.* Havana: Casa de las Américas, p. 197.

30 Agamben, G. (2006, 2015) *¿Qué es un dispositivo?* Barcelona: Anagrama, pp. 23–24.

31 Agamben, G. *Op. cit.* p. 24.

32 Idem, p. 27. See also: Agamben, G. (2005) *Profanaciones.* Barcelona: Anagrama, especially the text: "Elogio de la profanación", pp. 95–121.

33 Idem, p. 29.

34 Idem, p. 29.

35 Bachelard, G. (1970, 1985, 2012) *El derecho de soñar.* Mexico: FCE, pp. 105–106.

9

THE NEW VOIGHT-KAMPFF TEST AND DETECTING A *REPLICATING* SUBJECTIVITY

THE NEW VOIGHT-KAMPFF TEST
FOR DETECTING REPLICATING SUBJECTIVITY
IN GENETIC ANDROIDS.
FOUNDATIONS, APPLICATION and ACTUALISATIONS.
THEORETICAL and OPERATING MANUAL.
(REDUCED VERSION)
TYRELL CORPORATION.[1]

Module A. Generalities

Historical context and current situation. Basic concepts.
Test subjects. Fundamental objective

- According to the information available in Official Archives,[2] it was during the *Terminal World War* that the first Humanoid Robots known as *Synthetic Freedom Fighters* were utilized as a combat resource. That war ended thanks to a peace accord signed in the final moment before damage would have been irreversible. Of course, the partial destruction of the planet, the post-nuclear darkness in various geographic areas, frequent radioactive rains, and the extinction of thousands of animal and vegetable species soon spurred the economic recovery and accelerated expansion of *Integrated Global Capitalism*[3] that exponentially increased the need for massive emigration and

DOI: 10.4324/9781003129295-9

interplanetary colonization, so the design and fabrication of the soldier Humanoid Robots were modified and the first Organic-Genetic Androids, known simply as *Genetic Androids*, were produced.

• Capable of functioning in strange and hostile environments, endowed with medical knowledge and competencies, and full dominion of several languages, these organic-humanoid machines (that came to be known commonly by the nickname "skin-jobs")[4] soon became a fundamental resource for the massive emigration and interplanetary colonization programme due to the crucial support they offer in military, industrial, and civil fields, in labours that run from working as personal servants to performing as tireless peasants or highly-qualified workers, not to mention the option of offering their owners or administrators all manner of sexual services. In this way, the *Tyrell Corporation* has stimulated unprecedented economic growth by becoming integrated as an axis of the neo-colonial-industrial-interplanetary system.[5]

• In accordance with the *Post-War Law*, all colonists enjoy the right to receive, free of charge, (at least) one (civil) Genetic Android for the support and development of their activities upon relocating to and settling in the territory, for exploiting and holding dominion over materials and environmental resources, and for deploying accelerated strategies of socioeconomic consolidation. Genetic Androids must be delivered fully equipped and with a guarantee of loyalty. All this constituted a key incentive for private individuals and several corporations and businesses to offer transport services to the extra-terrestrial colonies.

• Pursuant to the foregoing, remaining on Earth will become increasingly difficult because the depauperisation of the ecology and health conditions imply the possibility of being classified as "biologically unacceptable" (that is, as a *special subject*), which means living virtually on the margins of history. Despite this, many people refused to emigrate, so large cities and suburbs on Earth, despite the ever-present cloud of dust that moves through numerous continental and oceanic areas and the multiple forms of social disintegration, have maintained an intense economic activity of production, circulation, and consumption of both modified or substitute foods, and diverse material, spiritual, and artistic goods that endure, fragmentarily, in the practices of daily co-existence, predominantly nocturnal in nature. Hundreds of thousands have remained grouped together, above all in urban zones (that are growing excessively), in spite of the very real possibility of having to change their area of residence according to the indices of variation of the toxic rains and the (always precarious) options of minimally-remunerated work.

- Even in the social contexts just described, the subjectivity of the population could be graded as *relatively sane*[6] though it is well-known that towards the virtually desolate suburbs one encounters extremely peculiar beings, like the intriguing case of the *special* John Isidore who "loved all living things, above all, animals", and from the age of sixteen devoted himself secretly – and against all local regulations – to a compulsion to resuscitate any dead animal he came upon.[7] Over time, the Government succeeded in regularizing distinct genetic tests for the residents who remained on Earth as a means of detecting emerging alterations, and other tests designed to determine minimal mental faculties; all with the objective of identifying, evaluating, relocating, and, if necessary, isolating dysfunctional individuals and those that posed the greatest social danger.

- The most severe problem of social control (in both the new spaces in the process of colonization and on Earth) emerged when the Genetic Androids, fundamentally destined to work in the interplanetary colonies, in a way incomprehensible to the established programming schemes, and despite enhanced cerebral units, began to escape from their respective activity centres by arbitrarily neutralizing all the localization devices in the network, and at times resorting even to physical violence against their owners or the personnel of the maintenance, review, and/or repair agencies involved, in order to flee using the multiple transportation circuits available and conceal themselves in distinct intermediate stations or even make their way back to Earth and pass themselves off as genuine biological subjects, either *normal* or *special*. The initial incident was a bloody riot by a team of Genetic Androids in a space colony in November 2019.[8] Since then, those organic machines are prohibited from remaining on Earth under penalty of death (in their case called *retirement*), unless they have specific authorization. The models involved in this systemic rupture are those of the T-14 and Nexus 6 series (provided their cerebral units have enormous technical development). From that juncture – and the alteration of functions that characterized it – forward, a transgression of the fundamental sense of service and productivity took hold, such that the aforementioned Genetic Androids (now converted, by virtue of their escape, in *Rebel* Genetic Androids) were conceived and constructed.

- Previously, the key indicator for differentiating between a Genetic Android and a genuine biological subject (aside, of course, from chemical analyses of bodily fluids and micro-surgical procedures to explore and verify codes) consisted in confirming their (up to then presumed) incapacity for any empathetic connection, understood as the absence of the "ability to *appreciate* the existence of other beings".[9] In the beginning, this ability could only be found in human communities of genuine biological subjects.[10] This approach was based on the idea that empathy is constituted as a faculty whose production requires an implicit gregarious propensity, psychosocial and political in nature, linked to eventual practices of solidarity that favour the subsistence and continuity of groups over time. Such a gregarious tendency made no sense in the programmes of the Genetic Androids designed for individual conservation and maintenance as service units and efficient multimodal functionality according to the goal of their fabrication.

- Such a solitary, self-sufficient organism, with structured functions, has no use for empathy. Indeed, this could become a factor of inefficiency in the fulfilment of its obligations. Following this logic, and given the need to locate and eliminate deviated cerebral units with great precision, Johann Voight designed a first instrument called "The Voight Test" (modified three years later by Lurie Kampff),[11] that was originally considered capable of detecting the Genetic Androids' inability to generate empathy or, perhaps better, the flattening of affect or the incapacity of animic fusion of an interpersonal character.

- The original Voight-Kampff Test, like some advanced polygraph instrument, consisted of 120 questions (100 base, 20 reserve); a pupil viewer or ocular scanner with its panel of indicators; a *smell fear* device; and an electronic chronometer. By analysing the meticulous recordings of reaction and response times to the test questions, and based on the parameters of biologically genuine subjects, the pupil viewer or ocular scanner was designed to measure ranges of "capillary dilatation in the facial region" and detect an eventual *blushing* reaction. Concretely as well, it had to register "tension in the eye muscles". The underlying assumption was that in the presence of a "morally disquieting" stimulus (materialized in any question on the instrument) the test would provoke an "autonomous, primary response" in human subjects linked to what was called as "shame" or "blushing"[12] that, moreover, could occur in relation to *sentimentally accentuated complexes*.[13] These reactions, it was believed, could not be controlled voluntarily (as can occur with such physiological indicators as breathing or heartbeat). Although in strictly biological terms these facial reactions and movements of the eye muscles could occur spontaneously in Genetic Androids, the test posited – based on laboratory experiences – that the test questions-stimuli (or *of induction*) would not provoke these reactions in them, confirmed by the ranges of measurement signalled by the needles of the indicators. The *smell fear* device functions by capturing floating particles associated with *fear* that emanated from subjects (in the case of *Rebel Genetic Androids*, conceived as a self-protection response to the objective threat of being intentionally *retired*); that is, this apparatus could "breathe" and biochemically process the test subject's smells in situations of real danger or risk for its processes of self-conservation and, in this way, ratify diagnoses.

- Experts were well aware, of course, that the Voight-Kampff Test was not infallible, but the true conflict arose when, with ever-greater clarity and frequency, *Rebel Genetic Androids* developed the capacity to pass the test, which thus lost all its reliability. Test administrators discovered that during application, capillary dilatation reactions and normal contractions of the iris muscle were produced in the facial region, the floating particles of fear ceased to be emitted, and, in the subjective domain of the test, *sentimentally accentuated complexes* came to be recognized clearly. Having successfully defeated the Test, the *Rebel Genetic Androids* became entities capable of producing signs of empathy and complex expressions of subjectivity absolutely unknown up to that time and, therefore, became able to consummate the delight of escape and the ability to pass as genuine biological subjects.

- This situation made it necessary to undertake a theoretical-methodological recomposition of the Voight-Kampff Test. Compared to the original version, the *New Voight-Kampff Test* introduces several modifications: 1) it eliminates as useless both the viewer (ocular scanner) and the *smell fear* device; 2) it reduces the number of questions-stimuli (various original questions remain, but new inductor elements were designed to integrate a questionnaire well-adapted to the unexpected complexities of the detection tasks to be performed); and 3) four new fixed sections (or series) of enquiry and testing were added to be applied when necessary, utilizing minimal materials and equipment. In general, the new version of the *Test* provided technicians, verification agents, psycho-engineers, judicial functionaries, and/or *Blade Runners* with greater flexibility of interpretation and analysis of the results before establishing diagnoses. *The fundamental turn of the new Test consists in that the object of enquiry is no longer the presence or absence of the capacity for empathy per se but, rather, the emergence of empathetic processes in the Android linked con-substantially to insubordination and the formation of groups and collectives of anticolonial indiscipline* (that is, processes linked to transgressing and/or re-creating the schemes of the individual programme implanted in each unit by the corporate design for work in the colonies), *through the emergence and articulation in the micro-political domain of an intense affective implosion and discourses and practices of a subversive and solidary character* (especially, for example, the exercise of *flight* in groups), *associated with imaginative expressions of transforming, existentially reinventing, and fracturing the established orders of functionality characteristic of any rebel subject.*

- When a Genetic Android produces detectable expressions of in-subordination, such as the instant of flight and desertion; that is, when it becomes a *Rebel Genetic Android* (and only at that moment), it shall be catalogued as a *Replicant*. Here, precision is highly significant: we can speak of a *Replicant* when a Genetic Android, from its arti-ficial condition as a functional copy or reproduction (that is, a replica) subject to pre-determined programming codes, suddenly becomes an entity that escapes, that produces unsuspected subjectivity, and that surpasses its reproductive condition of functioning sufficiently to generate an active character of its own with autonomous processes of reflection, intense affectivity, and ethical, aesthetic, and political behaviour. This implies an exercise or gesture of insubordination in word and act that involves, tacitly or explicitly, an objection to, criticism of, or protest against the existential orderings of origin, thus leading to the appearance in those Androids of an unpredictable, dangerous creative plexus that must be deactivated at all costs. The whole set of subjective expressions characteristic of *Rebel Genetic Androids*, or *Replicants*, shall be catalogued as *Replicant Subjectivity*. The fundamental objective of the *New Voight-Kampff Test*, then, is to opportunely detect *Replicant Subjectivity* in test subjects in order to determine their elimination; that is, or immediate *retirement*.

Module B. Diagnosis

Identification and descriptive analysis of replicant subjective expression. Programming alterations. Reduction or absence of self-controls. Systemic malfunctioning

- Replicant subjectivity is an expressive condition, emergent and dy-namic in character that never crystallises in fixed, immobile, or structural elements. Hence, a Genetic Android may be a *Replicant* today but not tomorrow. It may also transpire that a *Rebel Genetic Android* disintegrates replicant subjectivity only to later multiply it in other, unexpected replicant subjectivities; that is, an Android could produce replicant subjectivity (at different moments of its existence) and, of course, later articulate expressions and actions in consequence of this (that, in turn, will have distinct social and individual repercussions), though always through processes that could be classified as intermittent and distinct. It has yet not been possible to explain and characterize the reasons for which replicant subjectivity is produced and manifested in terms of such variable discontinuity. This does not mean that there is any weakness in the eventual dynamic integration of replicant subjectivity, for we speak of "a powerful subjectivity synthesized out of fusions of exterior identities and in the complex political-historical stratifications of its 'biomythography'".[14] In any case, the situation described clearly entails a challenge for the consequent diagnosis and detection that the *New Voight Kampff Test* must assume. Due to its very nature, replicant subjectivity will have multiple and diverse forms of specific constitution, which could bring together, in infinite combinations, the various indicators, features, or processes described in this *Theoretical and Operating Manual*. Therefore, during the application of the *New Voight Kampff Test* it will suffice for the police agents, technicians, judicial functionaries, or *Blade Runners* assigned, localise, to discover, encounter, or recognize *only one* of the lines of systemic malfunctioning, reduction, or absence of self-controls, and/or programming alterations, in order to immediately proceed with the retirement from circulation of the *Rebel Genetic Android* so detected.

• Replicant subjectivity implies diverse, intense processes of de-subjection and/or de-identification with respect to the original configuration patterns linked to corporate power. These processes of rupture or fragmentation bring the Android, in effect, close to the territory of abjection. In this logic, every *Replicant*, at some moment of its expression, betrays itself, goes back on its word, breaks down, negates itself, because by fracturing the subjection that is its basic constitution, it ceases to function in terms of pure subjection to establish (unforeseen) processes of the production of an alternate subjectivity, and because in this way it opens dynamics of change and transformation of the existential and interactive plexuses that surround it. "'Subjection' is the process of becoming subordinated to power, as well as the process of becoming a subject".[15] That is to say,

the primary identity of the Android as subject of service and functionality can only be configured through an original subordination to
corporate ordering materialized as power; ordering that introjects the
Android by means of the cognitive-behavioural and linguistic programmes it reproduces and without which all meaning of its existence perishes. This must occur in such a way that any Genetic
Android must form its own conscience, though always associated
with a kind of functional self-censure, effectuating the transmutation
of corporate values and interests in their most intimate psychic reality.[16] With the advent of rebelliousness, however, what happens is
that a sudden fracture of introjected power is produced by virtue of
which the android subject, through a passionate shift,[17] turns upon
itself, constitutes itself as a force that runs against the grain of its own
previous trajectory of effective functional articulation; thus establishing, ambivalently, a tragic exclusion or erasure of itself.

• The unforeseen self-configuration of the *Rebel Genetic Android* is
lived and realized by means of an intensification of affective reliefs,
which are projected as a superlative existence or *hyper-existence* that,
in truth, establishes links of productive searching not only with
ethical-political domains, but also, and very significantly, aesthetic
ones. Replicant subjectivity invents, for example, discursive lines and
practices of artistic variation to the previously established codified
platforms of personality, even when this outburst means a certain
transgression and a certain absurdity in relation to the networks of
efficient communication and interaction marked and utilized beforehand. Those discursive-sentimental lines of variation are detected
because they often include a useless beauty or something like apparent expressive nonsense; images or metaphors juxtaposed with the
functional components articulated in the corresponding network of
co-existence.[18] The *hyper-existence* or affective intensification of
Replicants and their derived expressions occur because their own
energy sub-systems have a flaw that leads them to generate an excess
of potency (*potentia*). All *potentia* is definable, in principle and in the
strict sense, by its opposition to the *act*, but at the same time, by
constituting itself as an "unstoppable tension to realisation" or, perhaps better, an "urgency towards the act".[19] And it is because
pleasure can occur only through the *act* that this, in turn, is converted
into a factor of unfulfillment of obligations. Thus, pleasure "is that
whose form is realised at each moment, that is perpetually in act".[20]
This means that the tension (anxiety, pain) of potency is relieved in
the moment at which one passes to the act. The role of corporate

power and its programmes (*potestas*) is precisely that of organizing and regulating, in a functional and adequate manner (through the previous introjection and incorporation of the corresponding mandates and orderings in Genetic Androids), the relation between potency and act. Thus, when the hypertrophy of the excess of potency arises in Androids and the lines of prescription or order-word implanted disintegrate or deteriorate, corporate power must appeal to the fundamental and originary power of isolating or separating in the *Replicants* the potency of their acts[21]; that is, the mission to control, decrease, or eliminate the potency by impeding, in consequence, both the eclosion of pleasure and its effects of affective intensification and disobedience in the cybernetic organisms.

• In opposition to what, in programmatic terms and those of corporate design, is catalogued as the *Inert Subjectivity* of the Genetic Androids (a normalized, functional, majoritarily, or strictly reactive – that is, desirable – subjectivity), *Replicant Subjectivity* implies constant (though eventually discontinuous) processes of multiform rebelliousness, micro-political insubordination, and sporadic practices of revolt organized in groups or collectively. The emergence of a replicant subjectivity in Genetic Androids constitutes a complex phenomenon that carries with it a paradoxical condition: replicant subjectivity (sometimes called *controverted subjectivity*) and the excesses of potency that it produces can be the effect of an excision or rupture of the very line of initial subordination or subjection installed in the programming of the Androids. According to theory:

> The power that is the condition of the subject is, by necessity, distinct from the power that the subject is said to exercise. The power that gives origin to the subject does not maintain a relation of continuity with the power that constitutes *its potency*. When power modifies its statute, passing from being a condition of the potency to become 'the potency of the subject itself' (…) a significant and potentially enabling inversion is produced.[22] This imperfection can be called "enabling rupture"[23] and it forms a nucleus of the production of subjective *resistance* in the Genetic Androids associated with a kind of unsuspected appropriation of power.

• The replicant subject lives in a permanent *escape* from both the apparatuses of capture deployed by corporate power, and itself, with respect to fixed or inert forms of functioning and co-existence. This situation – which necessarily entails a certain vulnerability – tends to be lived ambivalently given that in its constant flight, the Android can experience affective implosions of euphoria/enthusiasm or angst/desperation. Instants of quietude appear sporadically and irregularly, above all in the provisional nodes or points of the circulation networks, at the moment of rest to prepare the re-commencement, when the Androids produce peaceful and beautiful *imaginative stays* that they tend to feel as *nostalgia for what was never lived*. But in any case, escape is soon reactivated in terms of an unstoppable distance from the psychosocial nucleus of original conformation; a nucleus that (due to the effect of said evasion of the subject) first proceeds to disintegrate or lose ontological and political consistency or solidity only, perhaps, to later reconstitute itself in different and fragmentary ways. Replicant subjectivity begins "on a plane of consistency that includes (...) the territorialised existential regions" but develops subversively in access to "deterritorialised immaterial universes" that it (replicant subjectivity) strives to convert into the object of individual and collective reappropriation.[24] That is to say, replicant subjectivity escapes from the regimes of inertia and functional corporate reproduction through "experimenting virtual possibilities"[25] that literally involve a reinvention of subjective life in movement.

• Replicant subjectivity tends towards a very profound feminine condition. All *Replicants* are constituted by a *woman-potency* that involves them in specific forms of relation with, and understanding of, the world.[26] It is the instant linked to *becoming-woman* understood not as an excluding opposition with respect to any masculine subject, but as an intense circular movement of molecular transformation that vindicates the attitudes and practices directed towards deterritorialising some mode of authoritarian existence or other. Hence, becoming-woman means, for *Replicants*, the tendency to deconstruct what they themselves signal as *phallic identities*, associated with the imposition of truths, paranoia, social exclusion, despotism, arbitrariness, or humiliation and, dismantling that form of majority, reactive, and dominant thinking. Becoming-woman opens a path as a subjectivity that is dispersed, interconnected, decentred, and that escapes from the ordering frameworks established so as to flow constantly; all of which does not impede but, rather, promotes in an unusual way its disposition to combat and withdraw from the imperatives of stability. It is all about "the active reinvention of a jubilantly discontinuous 'Ego', in opposition to the consistently melancholic being programmed by phallogocentric culture."[27]

Becoming-woman, in any case, seems to incorporate in the *Rebel Genetic Androids* the dimension of empathy and compassion as domains eventually determinant of their decisions and actions of resistance.[28] Becoming-woman means, as well, *becoming-world*.[29] Replicant subjectivity tends towards a kind of affective fusion with each and every expression of the cosmos.

- Replicant subjectivity is consubstantial with respect to the event of desire. By definition, desire implies the fracture of the programmatic iteration in course; thus, replicant subjectivity is founded as a synonym of unpredictability, shock, and deformation. Desire is the fundamental, necessary, and primal condition of the replicant subject. Desire is, for *Rebel Genetic Androids*, a vital affirmation, one of exhilaration, formed in the context of combat and flight. The *Rebel Genetic Android* becomes a *desiring* subject (that seeks to go out of its way for something) when it should remain installed "quietly within itself"[30] exclusively as a desirable subject. But its desire – and this must be understood very well by corporate agents due to the dangers it entails – cannot be explained by the scarcity, a shortage, or the emptiness of its existence or its movements; its desire is not a derivation from deficit but an expansion of vitality; a gradient of subjective-corporal energy; an impetus that opens fire on absence and deprivation. The replicant attitude is never one of indigence or abandonment, but of abundance, profusion in its linkages, at times even of an exuberant presence and an aristocratic eccentricity.

- *Rebel Genetic Androids* provoke the strategic rupturing of the *Law of existential gravitation*.[31] All social ordering requires that every subject assume the prescriptive character of reality as it is disposed by means of its own decrees. This necessary elevation and acceptance of codes of conduct and interaction (that, by the way, can generate, minoritarily, some afflictions or sadnesses or the like) marks a profitable, useful moment for the psychological stability of the subject and for the adequate functional organization of collectives and the lines of corporate expansion. The aforementioned *Law* formalises the obligation of every subject to adhere to the conditions of the installed reality and support its dictums; that is, the obligation of every individual to subject himself and assume reality in its own terms. It is recognized that the "pressure of reality", by virtue of its own gravitational centre or force of attraction, can demand enormous efforts of adaptation and energy outlays that come to be lived as diverse impositions in a context of anonymous needs and cruelties that, generally-speaking, that individual cannot (should not) evade.[32] Well then, *Rebel Genetic Androids* violate the *Law* because they more-or-less deliberately deny, disavow, and/or subvert socially-installed reality. In other words, they are in contempt of the gravitational mandate of the current centre of co-existence and established functions, which they call "faceless despotism of the real" or "tyranny of the real".[33] The problem becomes more acute because this attitude "soon irradiates a pure and anarchical subjectivity in the world (...). The liberty manifested of one involuntarily tends towards the potential of liberty for the rest (...)".[34]

- *Rebel Genetic Androids*, in their diverse contacts with sex and eroticism both conventional and atypical, become fierce lovers of the orgasm because they often experience it with an intensity truly unknown to any genuine biological subject. One of the most interesting effects of their alterations in programming and the reduction of self-controls lies in the reality of feeling the orgasm simultaneously as: A) a cosmic outburst of laughter and sadness from the very depths of the body; B) a solemn sensation of infinity through the palpitations of the flesh; C) a gleaming explosion of blood and memories; D) a heart-breaking tenderness of weeping and joy due to the beauty of the world; and E) a crepuscular convulsion of interplanetary music. Eventually, as well, during the experience of orgasm, *Rebel Genetic Androids* emit a visceral, mysterious scream (like the bellowing of a buffalo) that can take the form of an interminable howling or a more-or-less discontinuous honking. In other cases, upon reaching climax, a thick, sky-blue coloured liquid spills from the mouths of female Androids.[35] The instant of the orgasm often envelops the induction or reactivation of neuronal and animic connections that, once consolidated, support in the deviant cybernetic organism, the advent of love: a moment in which the sweetness and generosity of the replicant subject reaches – due to someone or something – indescribable levels of plenitude.

- Controverted subjectivity is marked by an endless journey not only due to the forced effect of its attitude of escape, but also because the adventures and open voyage are constituted, precisely, as the "possibility of leaving oneself to go towards *the other*".[36] leaving oneself to go towards an uncertain future even though this produces an uprooting that seems to put an end, beforehand, to spaces of familiarity. In their constant journeying, *Rebel Genetic Androids* participate in a certain way in the symbolic, pragmatic, and political dismantling of a socio-functional platform installed for the reproductive stability of the orders of corporate meaning. This is how, while travelling, all replicant subjects rewrite the original programmes and exercise a garbled, shameless reinvention of their surroundings. This is an irreverent geographic and inter-spatial movement that opens the way towards a kind of everyday re-creation of their own existence; one that implies, no doubt, that all *Rebel Genetic Androids* formulate on a daily basis questions concerning life, the cosmos, nostalgia, or love, that are of great sentimental urgency and transcendent vocation, but which can never receive a definitive answer. During any odyssey, in all replicant subjectivity the real world and the virtual world are superimposed or fused; lucidity and dream; thought and the passions; algorithmic condition and imaginative condition; critique and fiction. That is to say: the natural and the supernatural are articulated to simultaneously found all subversive existential plexuses. This means that any city or landscape or sidereal limit, no matter how unknown (or perhaps because of this), is always perceived as being joined to the irradiation of a sad, sweet magic that incorporates the most dissimilar affections and generates something like a devotion full of gratitude, but also of uncertainty, upon breathing and living each instant of its tragic exile. This is how replicant subjectivity, in a poetic turn born in the invisible, converts the country into an "interior country"[37] or into an interior city, or into an interior universe (of indescribable beauty), because with this it announces the rupturing of the technical channels of an external and dominant truth. In the face of corporate power of knowledges and regulations, the Rebel Genetic Android resists and takes refuge in the unreachable distance of its intimacy; that is, in the emotional abyss of its stellar landscapes.

- Replicant subjectivity is created through a particularly profound anticolonial turn. The thought and affective and political implications of its animic reality produce an opposition as radical as it is dangerous with respect to the corporate orderings of work in the colonies.[38] The existential status of the replicant subject is linked, from its very origins, to the rupture of colonial work and its projections, and the effects of socioeconomic and intersubjective homogeneity and coherence. *Rebel Genetic Androids*, in their programmatic dis-arrangements, impugn the corporation's natural right to usufruct and maintain at its disposal – in benefit of its own interests – the products of work activity and the labour of the cybernetic organisms (all of which it manufactured). At certain moments, replicant subjects have been heard to utter absurd words like: "We are a small genus of humans: we possess a world apart, fenced in by dilated seas, novel in almost all the arts and sciences".[39] As part of its systemic malfunctioning, the Genetic Android abandons, from one moment to the next, its nature as a *copy* and its fundamental profile, strictly reproductive, to elevate itself, through a display of singularity and extravagance, as a replicant subject capable of conspiring, of provoking distinct forms of insurrection (utilizing for this purpose the very codes, conceptual instruments, and competencies previously supplied by the corporation).

- The corporate design gives the Genetic Androids of the latest generations, from their initial activation, a store of memories that have the function of emotionally catalysing and administrating the store of often frustrating and intense recent experiences during their brief interval of useful live. This is a more-or-less diffuse, complementary series of memory implants constituted (illusorily) as support for an internal perception of continuity and integration of each one's presumed biographic trajectory, intended to facilitate the psychological and social control of the Genetic Androids themselves.[40] The problem is that when flaws arise in the systemic malfunctioning the cybernetic organism develops, thanks to vectors of desire and imagination, pronounced processes of a vital re-invention or re-creation of its implanted memory that lead to the generation of contents not recorded in its initial programming. The engendering of this inventive memory evidences the rupture of a de-subjection in the Android, who wields those unexpected contents as an axis of deliberate resistance against the corporate mandate or order-word of adscription, belonging, and programmatic pertinence. This alludes to the elaboration of a minoritarian, paradoxical memory that, to the beat of diverse interactions and emotivity, promotes a constant resignifying of experiences and testimonies. The replicant attitude reveals that, upon re-positing and re-creating the implanted memory, the *Rebel Genetic Android* adopts a posture that challenges what they have denominated the *tyranny of the past* granted by the corporation. Based on theory, it is understood that this attitude "strips the memory of its homologation to a fixed identity based on the subject of the majority".[41] The replicant subject breaks away from imperative, systemic, or monolithic memory to produce "counter-", alternative, poetic, or minoritarian memories.[42] What follows is an intuitive production of memories-experiences that is directed towards deterritorialising the subjective spaces and anchors linked to the capture or congelation of its existence. "Remembering in this way requires (…) the careful disposition of potentiating conditions that permit the actualization of affirmative forces".[43]

- An important subjective condition of the *Rebel Genetic Android* is a tendency to disobey or ignore when summoned by the voice of authority in the exercise of interpellation, or even to respond with insults or rebellious acts (rupturing its foundational discursive sub-ordination).[44] "From this perspective, interpellation (…) is also (…) a command to place itself on the side of the law (…) and ingress into the language of self-adscription – 'I am here' – by appropriating guilt".[45] However, upon being interpellated by the forces of order, the replicant subject tends not to recognize itself in that summoning and/or fails to accept the implicit subjection that is sought to be imposed on it from without, or the psychopolitical condition of the guilty subject, which can at times be erased completely from its operating system. Nonetheless, for the effects of detecting replicant subjectivity, what the authority can often usefully employ is *direct injurious interpellation*, which frequently makes it possible to induce a bellicose, confrontational response characteristic of a subjectivity that unfolds in rebellion. This way of acting by the *Rebel Genetic Android* is related to the possibility of an open, creative *de-regulation* of its own subjectivity in the form of disobedience and the outright rejection of its elemental codes of subjection and fear of death. The replicant subject desires to live freely, free of persecution, free of fear.[46]

• There is, finally, a set of more-or-less recognizable psychosocial and linguistic elements that permit detection of replicant subjectivity. This can be deployed coldly in specific contexts, and is made up of the following data: A) The replicant subject vindicates the political projection of singularity and, with this, of contradictions, imperfection, and unpredictable gesture. It establishes alliances and actions of group solidarity but also resorts to displays of self-affirmation with no limitations or squeamishness in their specificity. B) Replicant subjectivity leads to an overflowing of vitality by virtue of which it rejects the fear of death and struggle and admits no other option than that of triumphing in its striving to re-create its existential plexuses (hence, they must be imperiously withdrawn (retired) from circulation as soon as possible). C) All Rebel Genetic Androids tend to *speak* in an eccentric, or strange, manner. The speech of the replicant subject (for example, during free association on the psychoanalyst's couch) qualifies as a poetic and/or tragicomic speech, subversive and enigmatic in tone. D) Something similar occurs in the way it writes, as it often re-codifies and jumbles up the processes of communication and modes of thinking in order to escape from the prescriptions of corporate power. Something else that tends to occur is that when writing they mix or overlap terms from one language with those of another, generating diverse neologisms and grammatical errors that preclude any linguistic totality identifiable with homogeneous discourse. This derives in a distinct, altered, at times decontextualized, writing that is more-or-less contradictory, fictional, and intense in nature. E) In the face of its inevitable functional deactivation (that is, death), once the limited energy supply installed during fabrication is exhausted, the *Rebel Genetic Android*, through the production of unrepeatable subjective meanings, succeeds in re-converting the process of decay into something that allows it to grow, diversify, multiply, re-compose itself, to survive and advance in disorder and disconcert. This poses an even greater danger as it propagates activities of rupture with the established social organization. In any case, the replicant subject assumes its destiny and truth as an aperture of the soul. One of them has said: *I shall pull from my chest the bloody soul and blandish it in the wind as a banner.*[47] It lives lyrically, between flashes of pain and felicity that open an uncertain path and a world of adventure. It often appears to seek refuge in the internal universe, just like artists, distracted in the complexity of a sentiment that suffers for the immediate, but glows enthusiastically for the landscape profiled in the distance. It lives its life with avidity though at the same time saddened for everything that remains without being lived. It shares its words with lustre, but something always subsists that is not expressed. In the end, the dreams and yearnings it does not achieve, become "living stars in the far-off sky of language, whose constellations we can barely decipher".[48]

Module C. Application

General Warning

The most important precaution to be taken by the judicial officials, or *Blade Runners*, whose job it is to apply the *New Voight-Kampff Test*, is mandatory: they must be armed and prepared to shoot the subject (after she/he has passed through a security review) at any moment during the test procedure. The recommendation is to use one of the most reliable pistols available in commercial circuits; for example, a Glock 19, GSh-18, SPS (panther) with expansive SR12 bullets, a 9-millimetre XM17 Sig Sauer, a small *Skoda* machine gun,[49] or a powerful Smith & Wesson model 500 revolver. This measure is essential for preventing incidents like the one committed by the *Replicant* Leon Kowalski (Nexus 6 N6MAC41717) who shot the *Blade Runner* Dave Holden while he was applying the *Voight-Kampff Test* during his police investigation.[50] The various sections of the *Test* are autonomous, so they can be applied separately in the order that seems most convenient at the time, though the questions of the *Basic Interrogation* should be used in every instance. The identification, discovery, encounter, or recognition of *one sole* line of systemic malfunctioning, reduction, or absence of self-controls, and/or programmatic alterations – even before completing the test – is deemed sufficient for the official assigned to immediately proceed to retire the *Rebel Genetic Android* so detected from circulation.

Spatial, material, and organisational conditions for administering the Test

The ideal space for administering the *Test* is grey and cold, illuminated by a white light that recalls the sensation of being dead. Preferably it will be night-time or as evening begins to descend with a gloomy sun. An artificial bird will fly softly through the high-ceilinged chamber. Through the one dreary window, "a ruinous, empty, gigantic edifice" is visible[51] amid the exterior confines of penumbra and the clouds of post-nuclear dust. Outside, enormous lights and voices will spout publicity and, eventually, a filthy rain will begin to fall that never ends. On the marble table lie several sheets of paper; a photo of a beautiful, unknown, face; a bottle of whisky with three small glasses; an electronic screen; a piano; an apple; a pen for writing; a music box; and a china lamp. The enquiry may begin with any test section and pass to any other at any moment, even without completing the previous one. Replicant subjectivity can be detected when one least expects it.

Sections of the test

1. *Basic interrogation*[52]

    a. Respond to the following questions, statements, or social situations immediately and in a loud voice:

        • *It's your birthday and they give you a calfskin wallet. How do you react?*

        • You're in the library writing a speech on the importance of philosophy. Soft music is perceptible in the atmosphere, but from one moment to the next it increases in volume too loudly. In a flash, a half-naked boy jumps on your table with a rabbit in his hand and begins to dance frenziedly.

        • It's night and you're in the cafeteria of a very elegant hotel in the city. Suddenly, a young, attractive woman begins to photograph you again and again using an intense flash. She does not answer your questions.

- *You have a young son. He shows you his butterfly collection and a killing jar. What do you do?*
- You enter, alone, the antechamber of an enormous cave in an unfamiliar landscape. A few steps inside you discover a very old table and on it you find a recently-used electric saw spattered with fresh blood.
- *You're watching television. Suddenly, you realize that a wasp is crawling up your arm.*
- A little girl dressed in school clothes is crying and screaming before the door of an abandoned building. Seeing you, she kneels and clasps your legs, imploring desperately: Don't do it! No, please, no! Don't do it!
- *You're watching a play. A banquet is going on during which the guests are enjoying an aperitive of live oysters. The first dish consists of cooked dog.*
- There's a golden mirror in an empty salon. You approach the mirror to look and realize that the face reflected there is not yours. A stormy wind blows outside.
- *You're reading a magazine and encounter a photograph of a naked man. He is lying face-up on a beautiful, enormous bearskin. Your spouse likes the photo and hangs it on the bedroom wall.*
- A scarecrow out in the middle of a field is being pecked by a flock of crows. When they feel your presence, the crows turn towards you, in silence.
- *You're walking in the sand in a desert when you see a large tortoise turning on its shell being burned by the sun. It moves its feet in desperation but cannot turn itself over without your help. But you don't help it. Why?*
- On a clear day with a very beautiful blue sky you visit a lovely garden with a white table full of relatives and friends from your childhood. At one table you discover your deceased father, eating alone. He looks at you but doesn't recognize you. What do you say to him?
- *Describe in a few words all the good things that come to mind about your mother.*
- *A group of people are visiting a fishermen's wharf in a town. They're hungry and enter a restaurant. One of them orders lobster and the chef throws a live lobster into a pot of boiling water.*
- Right beside you, a policeman is beating an adolescent on the ground who screams in pain. You are armed at that moment.

- *You've rented a small log cabin in the mountains. The area is still exuberant. Inside the cabin there are old maps on the walls and a fireplace over which there hangs a deer's head with broad antlers. In that instant you realize that the deer's eyes are staring at you with tremendous hate.*

- Describe in a few words all the good things that come to mind about a torturer of women.

- *The person you love leaves you to have feverish sex with someone else. She/he could not care less about leaving you with the children you have. You soon discover that she/he shares obscene photos with mutual friends.*

- You're travelling in an airplane above the clouds and fall asleep in your seat. When you wake up the plane is completely empty but still flying. You look out at the horizon through the window and can only see a line of orangish light through the penumbra.

- Thousands of people fill the town square. They're all wearing very distinct colourful masks. You grab an axe and strike one of them splitting her/his head in two. Immediately you hear an inhuman, deafening whistle.

- *Someone invites you to visit their home. You're offered a drink. You see a large, red heart-shaped bed. The place is decorated with bullfighting posters. You approach to look. The person closes the door, comes towards your back, surrounds you with her/his arms and sticks her/his tongue in your ear.*

- A group of demonstrators dressed in pyjamas walks slowly around in circles outside a closed-down school. Silently, they hold in hand blank placards. Right beside them a dog is tied up barking rabidly and desperately struggling while spewing foam from its snout. The dog is about to work itself free.

- A young woman seated in a chair is forced to watch as a group of men with military helmets on their heads masturbate around her. One of them sees you coming and gestures for you to take your place and join in the fun.

- You're peacefully asleep in the early morning when, right outside your door, you hear someone, order through a loudspeaker very agitated: You! Yes, you! Come out! Come out immediately!

- You're walking past a stinky, far-off dump. There are little mounds of filth everywhere, toxic waste, and smouldering refuse. A little boy is crouching down scrabbling for something among the garbage; he finds a rotten apple and begins to eat it.

- Do you like to shove a dildo up your ass?
- You enter your house at night, exhausted, and turn on your bedroom light. You find a naked elderly woman with no teeth standing up and pissing on your bed. She's howling with laughter.
- You're hungry. You cut some slices of bread and from the bread there appear hundreds of insects that instantly invade your body and the walls.
- Your children become trapped in a destroyed vehicle that is about to explode. You want to open the locked door but can't remember the combination of the opening mechanism. Only a few seconds remain. Terrified, they're shouting at you from inside.
- You gaze upon a beautiful, white city from the heights of a hill. You can live there quite comfortably if you wish. But at that moment, two young people of extraordinary beauty invite you to accompany them to travel around the world, making love in a threesome and exploring new lands. What do you decide?
- In the street, you run into a corpulent motorcycle rider with black leather jacket and long beard. He is smearing huge amounts of strawberry jam all over his motorcycle. Upon seeing you, he smiles and moves his tongue lasciviously.

b. Comment on each one of the following statements in relation to your own reality. It is categorically prohibited to answer only YES or NO.

- My father always loved me.
- I live with an unextinguishable fire in my throat.
- I suddenly laugh and cry for no reason.
- I always lie.
- My body is penetrated by other components.
- I curse life.
- A blue torrent runs through my veins.
- The general acts like an imbecile.
- Happiness is for those who arrive late.
- My birthday wish is to be a woman.
- The law darkens the fall of the evening.

- Poetry spills into space.
- I'd love to be the pilot of a spaceship that travels through the planets.
- My soul moves alone through the world.
- My head aches like a metal day on the shoulders.
- Danger generates an indescribable pleasure.
- I can feel a terrible attraction for landscapes.
- I would do anything to change my name.
- I've never been able to kiss a horse's mouth.
- The police are after me.
- I can't concentrate on one sole thing.
- My memory has many truths to tell me.
- I want to break the window with a hammer.
- I never get tired of imagining a turtle.
- Yes, I believe that another world is possible.
- I'm receiving all the punishment of my years.
- I want to take a long trip over radioactive seas.
- Something is wrong with my existence.
- The beating of my heart illuminates the quietude of the firmament.
- I return to a place I have never known.
- I have rough sex with a pig.
- I feel like I'm a doomed person.
- My sweat is elegant.
- Sometimes I can't beat temptations.
- I know that my sins are unpardonable.
- They say I talk in my sleep.
- If I'd known you were coming I'd have baked a cake.
- I'm someone very sensible with cats.
- I often feel that clouds aren't real.
- Every time I speak, I'm assaulted by strangeness.
- Dying can't be all that bad.
- Sometimes I see the knife that cuts the poisoned meat.
- Someone must be controlling my thoughts.
- I detest it when people ask me personal questions.
- I'm scared of lightning.
- I keep myself intelligent beside the fire.
- I love to fight criminals.
- I admit that sometimes I should eat a little less.
- A great tension tears through my conversations.
- Some of my relatives have a bad character.

- I can't do anything well.
- For me, the future is bereft of hope.
- At this very moment, there are spiders climbing up a tree.
- I'd like to dress up as an admiral.
- *I love, though later I'm obligated to howl.*[53]

Criteria for detecting replicant subjectivity, Section 1: If as a result of any of the responses given by the subject there appears an insinuation, a brief argument, a furtive glance, a slip, a discreet startle, a failed expression, or some specific word, this will be considered sufficient to reveal (in the judgement of the official, or *Blade Runner*, in charge) the presence (more-or-less useful or explicit) of some alteration in the programming, a reduction or absence of self-control, or systemic malfunctioning (as described in this *Theoretical and Operating Manual*), and so verify a positive diagnosis. Categorically, if the subject mentions in any response one of the critical words listed below, this shall be considered immediate corroboration of its replicant or insubordinate condition. The critical words are: "daring"; "heart"; "desperation"; "voyage"; "gale"; "open sky"; "diamond"; "river"; "spring"; "city"; "imagination" and "sortilege".

2. *Interpretation of abstract images in movement*[54]

   a.   Freely express what it is you see in the following abstract images in movement:

   - *Denomination of image in movement 1:*
     A green island sustains its luminous pain through the night.
   - *Denomination of image in movement 2:*
     The tunnel of redemption leads conduces inexorably to your planet.
   - *Denomination of image in movement 3:*
     The ship of delirium goes away forever in silence.
   - *Denomination of image in movement 4:*
     The red bird dazzles with the invention of the constellations.
   - *Denomination of image in movement 5:*
     Your eyes cry for the dawn that will never return.
   - *Denomination of image in movement 6:*
     A face full of fury gives birth to memories that do not exist.
   - *Denomination of image in movement 7:*
     A desert holds your heart in the very centre of desperation.

- *Denomination of image in movement 8:*
  The solar beast awaits, erect, the arrival of the flowers.
- *Denomination of image in movement 9:*
  The fire withdraws due to the unpredictable display of music.
- *Denomination of image in movement 10:*
  Sadness dissipates upon travelling over the unspeakable backs of your hands.

Criteria for detecting replicant subjectivity, Section 2: In the subject's interpretation of the abstract images in movement, the indicators of emotional and corporal *control* must be monitored, together with *adjustment*, *maturity*, and *constriction* during the test situation; that is, if in the presence of the images shown on the screen the individual reveals unrest, any unjustified enthusiasm, or some form of hyperactivity, then we have before us a controverted subjectivity. With respect to its concrete responses, it is necessary to observe the categories of the *ubication* of the figure or object "seen"; the *content* of its elaboration, and the *determinant* aspects of such a response (that is, form, movement, texture, and colour). In inert subjectivity (which is desirable for the corporation), together with an attitude of control, adjustment, and maturity, one will observe responses that are centred, that have habitual content, and that are in equilibrium regarding the determinant elements. Any rupture, outburst, or excess of affect and imagination regarding the desirable response will be an unequivocal signal of rebelliousness. Having said this, for this section of the test there exists a series of critical expressions (or prototypical responses of subversive turn) that categorically evidence replicant subjectivity. These critical expressions (that can appear at any moment of the test) are as follows: "the ascending movement of a rabbit", "a hand fan of the rainbow", "hooded women as witches", "bodies that writhe inside the laboratory", "a self-absorbed ballerina", "blue crabs taking flight", "my grandmother's black, deformed dance", "clowns with hands held high", "electric butterflies filled with sadness", "my spaceship exploded into flashes of tenderness", "the inanimate movement of a mythological beast", "carnivorous flowers gnawing away at pride", "an explosion of scientific blood and lights", "the treasure map dissolving in time", "thousands of masks falling over a cliff", "an aristocrat shouting alone in the middle of the ocean", "elephants rolling upside down", "a human pelvis dancing the mambo of spite", "several young dogs juggling with something in their noses", "a green octopus trapping love with its tentacles", "many flags billowing in the spire of towers", "the goddesses of vengeance unleashing their fury against the cat", "a salamander and a kangaroo approaching the window", "attack angels bearing their hatred in the crepuscule", and "a giant tart slowly melting on nostalgia".

3. ***Production of fictitious stories base on stimuli***[55]

a. Based on the presentation of the following stimuli (images, objects, or words), narrate, for each case, a brief imaginary story:

Stimulus 1
Painting: "The Scream" by Edvard Munch.
Stimulus 2
An apple.
Stimulus 3
Photograph: "*Las Meninas (Autorretrato según Velázquez)*" by Joel-Peter Witkin.
Stimulus 4
Word: "Trembling".
Stimulus 5
A bottle of whisky.

Criteria for detecting replicant subjectivity, Section 3: The stories that the subject narrates must be interpreted, insofar as possible, in relation to previous specificities and knowledge of the case; but if the conditions for this do not exist, the interpretation *in vacuo* will also be valid. The stories must be evaluated in their *totality* but by exposing the *essential motives* that propel each one. At the same time, it is important to review the *dynamic sequence* and capture each significant datum in context (antecedent-motive-consequence); that is, to appraise the conditions, intensity, and consequences of the narration. Also to be considered are the story's *recurrences*, *concurrences*, and *interrelations*. Any decentring, rupture of the argumentative axes, enthusiasm, eccentricity, or unnecessary imaginary in the production of the stories constitutes a positive indicator of replicant subjectivity. In addition, however, there is a series of critical elements of the eventual narration (for any of the stimuli), whose enunciation will immediately prove the presence of controverted subjectivity. These critical elements are the following: "...a woman opens the door and finds the body of a loved one that has committed suicide", "...the spaceship crashes onto the beach, spilling tons of fresh, delicious fruit", "...a mad scientist wants to destroy the world but suffers because of his good daughter who loves him", "... Christ did not dare to reveal his liking for men", and "...a drunken young man is apprehended by the authorities beside a psychedelic lantern".

4. *Exercises of alteration of the human figure*[56]

  a. Draw a human figure that could be described as very attractive.
  b. Draw a human figure that could be described as monstruous.
  c. While looking at the following photographic portrait, take a marker and paint anything you want on its face and body.
  d. Write a poem with five verses on your own human figure (must include at least two metaphors of your genital organs).
  e. While listening to the music you are about to hear, dance in the freest and most open manner you can.

Criteria for detecting replicant subjectivity, Section 4: The replicant subject describes as a *monstruous* human figure the one associated with the context of the scientific, financial, and military institutions of the corporation; Well-conceived, homogeneous figures in efficient equilibrium with their surroundings. Any element that suggests a similar attitude in the corresponding drawing will be an unequivocal signal of a positive diagnosis. In addition, describing as a very *attractive* human figure one that includes any kind of eccentricity or rarity, no matter how subtle. In this sense, they tend to draw and describe as very attractive, human figures (prone to ontological and recreative hybridization) that pertain to peripheral contexts like the circus, fairground barracks, abandoned factories, autumn fields, imaginary zoos, nocturnal bordellos, or cold, far-away coasts. They establish a particular affective link with those models that theory defines as "dissidents of the universe",[57] such as the trapeze artist in her short dress of lights, the battered captain of a pirate ship, the accursed poet, the monkey woman or bearded lady, the philosophy student, or the *geisha* who strips silently. Regarding the instruction to alter the photograph with a marker, the key difference between inert and replicant subjectivity consists in that the latter does not trace (as any functional, well-adapted subject would) the previously established lines in the figure of the photo, but modifies them intensely, clearly, and surprisingly to generate, literally, an image quite distinct from the original one. Concerning the verses, the fundamental replicant characteristic will be a metaphorical overflowing and an evident enjoyment of writing; whereas with the request to dance in the freest most open way possible, the key aspect of the diagnosis will be the absence of traditional proxemic codes, such that, suddenly, the subject moves and agitates its hips and arms to the rhythm of the music like a madman who applauds and laughs with no regulation whatsoever, even offering, for moments, certain truly incomprehensible guttural noises.

5. *Direct insulting interpellation*

Note on a methodological warning: When the moment comes to apply this section of the test, the correct procedure consists in an exercise of offending the subject **without prior warning or explanation whatsoever**; using a tone of manifest hostility and disdain in an attempt to provoke the eventual appearance of a *replicant* response. The following expressions will be shouted almost directly in the subject's face in the order considered most effective according to each subject's particularities (adding others that the person applying the test prefers):

- Black piece of shit!
- Whore!
- Faggot!
- Asshole!
- Putrid slave!
- Skin-job!
- Leper!
- Indian imbecile!
- Pussy!
- Slut!
- Dike!
- Brown-noser!
- Piece of shit!
- *Motherfucker!*

Criteria for detecting replicant subjectivity, Section 5: As this *Manual* indicates, there comes a moment when replicant subjectivity, in contrast to the inert form, cannot resist emitting a more-or-less passionate contestation against *direct insulting interpellation*. This means that during the realization of this section of the test the insubordinate subject will eventually cede to the indignation produced in it by the provocative insults shouted at it. A functional, well-adapted Genetic Android will accept insults showing good self-control and serenity, and will not respond in kind. At most, it may timidly ask why it is being treated in such a manner. Thus, it is sufficient that the test subject react to any one of the expletives shouted by responding verbally or corporally with a gesture of rejection and combat for the examiner, or *Blade Runner*, to verify a positive diagnosis.

Final assurance

If after performing the complete process of *Test* application the legal official in charge holds any uncertainty regarding the final diagnosis, the corporate indication is that, in the interests and benefit of the established order, he proceed at that very instant and without second thought to fire his gun several times directly at the subject's chest. This will allow him to verify, whatever the case, that if the expansive bullets destroy a *Replicant's* chest and mix with the undecipherable couplings of the destroyed bio-machinery and blood that gushes forth, a blue sky full of moribund doves helplessly flapping their wings will appear.[58]

Perpetuity of the corporation

Final prescription (of an imperative and unappealable character): If the person who applies or studies the *New Voight-Kampff Test*, regardless of her/his position or technical-political functions, experiences or senses (albeit for just a fleeting moment) that she/he sympathizes, coincides, or connects with any of the alterations of the programming, the reduction or absence of self-controls, or systemic malfunctioning, she/he shall take her/his gun and silently, without further delay, shoot her/himself in the temple.

Notes

1 *Blade Runner: The final cut.* Directed by Ridley Scott, 2007.
2 Dick, Philip K. (1968) *¿Sueñan los androides con ovejas eléctricas?* Barcelona: Planeta DeAgostini, 2006.
3 See: Guattari, F. (2004) *Plan sobre el planeta. Capitalismo mundial integrado y revoluciones moleculares.* Madrid: Traficantes de sueños.
4 *Blade Runner: The final cut.* Directed by Ridley Scott, 2007, minutes 11:32 and 14:55.
5 Dick, Philip K. (1968) *¿Sueñan los androides con ovejas eléctricas?* Ed. cit. 2006, p. 54.
6 Idem, p. 27.
7 Idem, p. 34.
8 *Blade Runner: The final cut.* Directed by Ridley Scott, 2007, minutes 11:52 and 13:20–13:32.
9 Dick, Philip K. (n2) p. 52. Italics added.
10 Idem, p. 40.
11 Idem, p. 46.

12 Idem, p. 56.
13 See: Jung, C. G. (1934) "Consideraciones generales sobre la teoría de los complejos", *Obra completa. Volumen 8. La dinámica de lo inconsciente*. Madrid: Trotta, 2004, p. 101.
14 Haraway, D. (1991) *Ciencia, ciborgs y mujeres. La invención de la naturaleza*. Madrid: Cátedra, 1995, p. 299.
15 Butler, J. (1997) *Mecanismos psíquicos del poder. Teorías sobre la sujeción*. Madrid: Cátedra, 2001, p. 12.
16 Idem, p. 13.
17 Idem, p. 17.
18 See: *Blade Runner: The final cut*. Directed by Ridley Scott, 2007, minutes 1:32:40–1:33:22.
19 Agamben, G. (1985) *Idea de la prosa*. Buenos Aires: Adriana Hidalgo, 2015, p. 55.
20 Idem, p. 65.
21 Idem, p. 65.
22 Butler, J. (1997) *Mecanismos psíquicos del poder. Teorías sobre la sujeción*. Madrid: Cátedra, 2001, p. 23.
23 Ibid.
24 Félix Guattari cited by Braidotti, R. (2015), *Lo posthumano*. Barcelona: Gedisa, p. 112.
25 Ibid.
26 Deleuze, G.; Guattari, F. (1980) *Mil mesetas. Capitalismo y esquizofrenia*. Valencia: Pretextos, 2002. Especially, section 10: "1730 Devenir-intenso, devenir-animal, devenir imperceptible…" pp. 239–315.
27 Braidotti, R. (2004) *Feminismo, diferencia sexual y subjetividad nómade*. Barcelona: Gedisa, p. 172.
28 *Blade Runner: The final cut*. Directed by Ridley Scott, 2007, minutes 1:45:30–1:48:20.
29 See: Braidotti, R. (2009) *Transposiciones. Sobre la ética nómada*. Barcelona: Gedisa.
30 For the analysis of the notion of *desvivirse* (yearn for), see: Marías, J. (1984) *Breve tratado de la ilusión*. Madrid: Alianza, pp. 140–144.
31 See: Sloterdijk, P. (2017) *Estrés y libertad*. Buenos Aires: Godot, pp. 35–46.
32 Idem, p. 38.
33 Idem, pp. 38–39.
34 Idem, pp. 43–44.
35 See the film: *Hombre mirando al sudeste*, written and directed by Eliseo Subiela, 1986.
36 Birulés, F. (2000) Del sujeto a la subjetividad. Duro deseo de durar. In: Cruz, M. (Comp.) *Tiempos de subjetividad*. Barcelona: Paidós, pp. 223–234.
37 Expression of Edgard Mittelholzer, cited by Yanes, P.; Padrón, S. (2016) *Las poéticas visionarias*. Havana: Letras cubanas, p. 232.
38 *Blade Runner. The final cut*. Directed by Ridley Scott, 2007, minutes 11:52 and 13:20–13:32.
39 Words of Simón Bolívar in his "Carta de Jamaica" (1815), cited by Fernández Retamar, R. (2016) *Pensamiento anticolonial de nuestra América*. Buenos Aires: CLACSO/Casa de Las Américas, p. 141.
40 See: *Blade Runner. The final cut*. Directed by Ridley Scott, 2007, minutes 22:08–22:30.

41 Braidotti, R. (2004) *Feminismo, diferencia sexual y subjetividad nómade*. Ed. cit. p. 170.

42 The expression "*contramemoria*" (counter-memory) is from Michel Foucault (1971) *Nietzsche, la genealogía, la historia*. Valencia: Pretextos, 2004, p. 63.

43 Braidotti, R. *Ob. cit.* p. 171.

44 See: Althusser, L. (1970) Ideología y aparatos ideológicos del estado. In: *La filosofía como arma de la revolución*. Mexico: Pasado y presente, 1980, pp. 97–141. Especially the epigraph, "Ideology interpellates individuals as subjects", pp. 130–134.

45 Butler, J. (1997) *Mecanismos psíquicos del poder. Teorías sobre la sujeción*. Madrid: Cátedra, 2001, p. 120. The complete Chapter 4 can be reviewed due to its importance: "La conciencia nos hace a todos sujetos. La sujeción en Althusser", pp. 119–145.

46 *Blade Runner. The final cut*. Directed by Ridley Scott, 2007, minutes 1:45:10–1:45:18.

47 Paraphrase of the verses by Vladímir Mayakovsky. A more literal translation would be: "When the onset of the insurrection is announced, / and they go out for the encounter of the saviour's year, / I shall take out my soul for you, / I shall open it so as to make it larger, / and bloodied I shall raise it as a flag." See: (1915) *La nube en pantalones*. Mexico: Grijalbo Mondadori, 1999.

48 Agamben, G. (1985) *Idea de la prosa*. Buenos Aires: Adriana Hidalgo, 2015, p. 72.

49 *Skoda* machine guns are mentioned specifically in Dick, Philip K. (1968) *¿Sueñan los androides con ovejas eléctricas?* Barcelona: Planeta DeAgostini, 2006, p. 51.

50 *Blade Runner. The final cut*. Directed by Ridley Scott, 2007, minutes 4:50–7:22.

51 Dick, Philip K. (1968) *¿Sueñan los androides con ovejas eléctricas?* Barcelona: Planeta DeAgostini, 2006, p. 25.

52 The many questions, statements, and imaginary social situations presented in this section of the *Test* were composed under the influence of ideas from various sources. For sub-section a, the *Items* written in Italics were taken, with brief variations, from both Dick, Philip K.'s work (1968) *¿Sueñan los androides con ovejas eléctricas?* Barcelona: Planeta DeAgostini, 2006, pp. 59–62, and the film *Blade Runner. The final cut*, Directed by Ridley Scott, 2007, minutes 4:50–7:22 and 19:43–21:18. The other elements emerged from variations on distinct proposals in *Happenings* y *Performances*. See: Kaprow, A. (2013) *Ensayo sin título y otros happenings*. Mexico: Tumbona. See also: V.A. (n/d) *Perder la forma humana. Una imagen sísmica de los años ochenta en América Latina*. Madrid: Museo Nacional Centro de Arte Reina Sofía, Ministerio de Educación Cultura y Deporte. And finally, Taylor, D.; Fuentes, M. (Eds.) (2011) *Estudios avanzados de performance*. Mexico: Fondo de Cultura Económica. For sub-section b, some of the elements presented are inspired in questions from the well-known Minnesota personality inventory. See: Butcher, J. N.; Graham, J. R.; Ben-Porath, Y. S.; Tellegen, A.; Dahlstrom, W. G. and Kaemmer, B. (2019) *MMPI-2. Inventario Multifacético de Personalidad de Minnesota-2* (4th Ed.) (adapted by A. Ávila-Espada and F. Jiménez-Gómez). Madrid: TEA.

53 Aragon, L. (1931), fragment of the poem "Licantropía contemporánea" in: *Persecuté Persecuteur* Paris: Stock, 1998.

54 The design of this section of the *Test* is inspired in the work of *LIQUID-DO Interactive audio-visual performance*, which explicitly suggests the possibility of its

use as a projective technique in psychological diagnostics. See the proposal at: https://vimeo.com/26627213 Also reviewed were photographs from the *Abstract Artist Gallery* at https://www.abstractartistgallery.org/main-gallery/, especially the work of Mike & Madeleine Bülow. Of course, the idea of interpreting abstract images for clinical psychodiagnostics originated with Rorschach, H. (1921) *Psicodiagnóstico. Una prueba diagnóstica basada en la percepción.* Mexico: Manual Moderno, 2000. In this regard, in designing the interpretative categories I also found it useful to review: Klopfer, B.; Kelly, D. (1996) *Técnica del psicodiagnóstico de Rorschach.* Mexico: Paidós and Bohm, Y. (1953) *Manual del Psicodiagnóstico de Rorschach.* Madrid: Morata, 1973. Additionally: Pardillo, J.; Fernández, P. (2001) *Psicodiagnóstico de Rorschach. Un manual para la práctica.* Camagüey: Ácana. And, finally, Bar Din, A. (2001) *La test de Rorschach. Un manual de aplicación pluricultural.* Mexico: Siglo XXI, 2012.

55 This section of the test was conceived under the influence of Murray, H. A.'s classic projective instrument (1935) *Test de apercepción temática (TAT). Manual para la aplicación.* Buenos Aires: Paidós, 1977.

56 The fundamental antecedent for conceiving this section of the test in subsections a, b, and c, is, of course, found in Machover's extremely important test of the human figure. See: Portuondo, J. A. (2007) *Test proyectivo de Karen Machover: la figura humana.* Madrid: Biblioteca Nueva. Sub-sections d and e evoke some exercises of psychodramatic intervention. See: Moreno, J. L. (1987) *Psicodrama.* Buenos Aires: Hormé, and: Ramírez, J. A. (1987) *Psicodrama. Teoría y práctica.* Mexico: Diana.

57 See: Amara, L. (2013) *Los disidentes del universo.* Mexico: Sexto Piso.

58 The expression "moribund doves" comes from the poem "El holandés Cristián Huitman" by Federico García Lorca. The original verse reads: "*I would like to see you opened up / to see your moribund doves*". See: Arias de la Canal, F. (2001) *Antología de la poesía homosexual y cósmica de Federico García Lorca.* Mexico: Frente de Afirmación Hispanista, p. 104.

ANNEX 1

PHOTOGRAPH BY JOEL-PETER WITKIN ENTITLED *"LAS MENINAS (AUTORRETRATO SEGÚN VELÁZQUEZ)"* (1987)

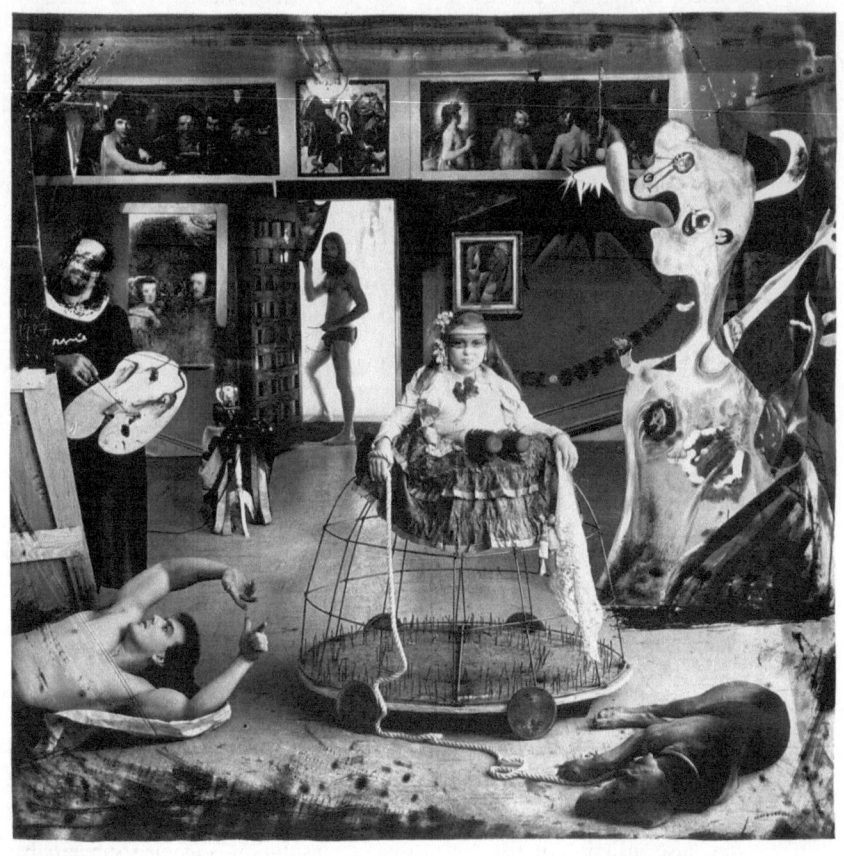

INDEX